A Practitioner's Guide and Data Protection

A Practitioner's Guide to Cybersecurity and Data Protection offers an accessible introduction and practical guidance on the crucial topic of cybersecurity for all those working with clients in the fields of psychology, neuropsychology, psychotherapy, and counselling.

With expert insights, it provides essential information in an easy-to-understand way to help professionals ensure they are protecting their clients' data and confidentiality, and protecting themselves and their patients from cyberattacks and information breaches, along with guidance on ethics, data protection, cybersecurity practice, privacy laws, child protection, and the rights and freedoms of the people the practitioners work with. Explaining online law, privacy, and information governance and data protection that goes beyond the GDPR, it covers key topics including: contracts and consent; setting up and managing safe spaces; children's data rights and freedoms; email and web security; and considerations for working with other organisations.

Illustrated with examples from peer-reviewed research and practice, and with practical 'top tips' to help you implement the advice, this practical guide is a must-read for all working-from-home practitioners in clinical psychology, developmental psychology, neuropsychology, counselling, and hypnotherapy.

Catherine Knibbs, NCPS, is a UKCP Child/Adult Psychotherapist with a background in technology, research, and practice. She is an Online Harm Consultant, Educator, Author, TEDx Speaker, and Child Safety Advocate in the world of technology. She is the director of Privacy4 and Catherine Knibbs Ltd.

Gary Hibberd is a Cyber Security Consultant with over 27 years in the industry. Gary is an expert in information security, cyber security, and data protection, helping organisations large and small to make sense of their security processes and practices such as ISO 27001, ISO 27701, and ISO 22301.

A Practitioner's Guide to Cybersecurity and Data Protection

How to Ensure Client Confidentiality

Edited by
Catherine Knibbs and Gary Hibberd

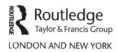

LONDON AND NEW YORK

Cover image: © Getty Images

First published 2024
by Routledge
4 Park Square, Milton Park, Abingdon, Oxon OX14 4RN

and by Routledge
605 Third Avenue, New York, NY 10158

Routledge is an imprint of the Taylor & Francis Group, an informa business

British Library Cataloguing-in-Publication Data
A catalogue record for this book is available from the British Library

Library of Congress Cataloging-in-Publication Data
Names: Knibbs, Catherine, editor. | Hibberd, Gary, editor.
Title: A practitioner's guide to cybersecurity and data protection : how to ensure client confidentiality / edited by Catherine Knibbs and Gary Hibberd.
Description: Abingdon, Oxon ; New York, NY : Routledge, 2023. |
Includes bibliographical references.
Identifiers: LCCN 2023018718 (print) | LCCN 2023018719 (ebook) |
ISBN 9781032427591 (hardback) | ISBN 9781032427607 (paperback) |
ISBN 9781003364184 (ebook)
Subjects: LCSH: Computer security. | Data protection.
Classification: LCC QA76.9.A25 P744 2023 (print) | LCC QA76.9.A25
(ebook) | DDC 005.8--dc23/eng/20231012
LC record available at https://lccn.loc.gov/2023018718
LC ebook record available at https://lccn.loc.gov/2023018719

ISBN: 978-1-032-42759-1 (hbk)
ISBN: 978-1-032-42760-7 (pbk)
ISBN: 978-1-003-36418-4 (ebk)

DOI: 10.4324/9781003364184

Typeset in Galliard
by Taylor & Francis Books

Contents

Figures

Foreword

I was delighted to hear from Cath and Gary that they were putting together this book. Becoming comfortable and confident with data protection, and having a solid understanding of the reasons why it's actually vital to do so, is something that could do with bringing to the forefront of the profession.

Having worked at the National Counselling & Psychotherapy Society (NCPS) for over eight years now, I know first-hand how overwhelming and worrying many therapists find all things to do with GDPR and data protection. I feel that this is the reason that practitioners are scared to engage with it; but that once they have even a basic understanding of it, suddenly they'll realise the implications and actually feel compelled to *do something* about it. Honestly, I find it daunting, too, which is why I think it's important to know where to go for advice and expertise. There are so many things that need to change once you realise the extent to which data *isn't automatically* protected by the technology we've grown to trust, and the systems we've built for ourselves to make our lives easier.

I've known Cath and Gary for a number of years now, and when I first met them in the height of the COVID pandemic via a (then) very modern and *de la mode* Zoom meeting, I was comforted by the depth of knowledge and experience that they both exuded, and the confidence with which they could talk about the subject of privacy, security, and data protection, answering all my questions with clarity and kindness. Having mentioned them to colleagues in the profession, those who know them speak very highly of them.

As time has gone on, and I've gotten to know them both better, I can safely say that this is their passion. Every conversation I have with Cath adds another wrinkle to my brain in terms of data protection, the safety of clients, and what best practice actually looks like. It's clear that Gary lives and breathes cybersecurity, and is doing everything in his power to make sure everyone knows how vital it is.

I recall, before I went on maternity leave in 2018, looking into what the NCPS's responsibilities were regarding GDPR, and I implemented some new processes and procedures for the Society. I attended meetings, lectures, and seminars on the subject; I read hundreds of pages of government guidance, and the same amount in easier-to-read guidance. My GDPR folder was by far and away the most overstuffed folder on my cabinet. I was thoroughly immersed in the world of GDPR for a short while, and naturally continued to keep up to date and refresh my mind on legislation to make sure we're always doing what we should be doing. All this is to say that I know how important it is.

Back when I first started learning about it, though, there wasn't anything straightforward, or that told me what I actually needed to know; even the easier-to-read guidance could be formidable. Perhaps that was because it was new to *everyone*, and everyone was, maybe secretly, just a tiny bit overwhelmed by it too. There wasn't anything that said: 'Hey, I understand this – here, let me explain it to you.'

I truly believe that you can only explain something in simple terms to someone else when you understand it yourself. Cath and Gary *are* adept at explaining all the important things you need to know in simple and accessible terms; that tells me that they really know what they're talking about. If you consider this alongside their massive amount of experience in this area, then I'm sure you'll also come to that same conclusion.

The people that they've called on to contribute to this book are all people *they* trust to share their wisdom with you, which is really saying something. If Cath and Gary trust you to talk about data protection, privacy, and security so much that they'll put it in a book? Well, the rest of us can be confident in trusting you, too.

So, my advice is this: read this book, use it to better understand data protection and security to make sure your practice is compliant, and be reassured that you've taken the best advice from people you can trust.

This guide will be a *vital* resource for anyone in the talking therapies professions. We hold some of the most protected data there are: vulnerabilities, secrets, and fears, and we should all be making sure that we treat that data with the care and respect they deserve, both legally and morally.

Thank you, Cath and Gary, for bringing together this book, the contributors for writing it, and my very best wishes to everyone using this guide to enhance their practice.

Meg Moss
National Counselling & Psychotherapy Society,
Head of Policy & Public Affairs

Acknowledgements

Gary and Cath want to dedicate this book to the contributors and thank them for their patience with the nagging that has taken place from Cath over the last five years. Thank you for the time and effort you have put into the book production, including those emails Cath kept sending you! Your patience has not gone unnoticed.

Further thanks go to the organisations who have supported this work and the book and the National Counselling & Psychotherapy Society's unwavering support via Meg Moss.

Gary would like to personally thank his wife for the support she provides on a daily basis.

Cath would like to thank Gary for the last five years of friendship and support in this domain (and for repeatedly answering questions), and for providing his time for those evening video calls during lockdown to the attendees of the Privacy4 course. I believe the ones who turned up benefited greatly from the advice and guidance you gave in the domain of data protection and cybersecurity. Thank you for your time and passion here in this book.

Additional author biographies

Maria Bada is a Lecturer at Queen Mary University in London. Maria is a behavioural scientist whose work focuses on the human aspects of cybersecurity and cybercrime. Her research looks at the effectiveness of cybersecurity awareness campaigns trying to identify factors that potentially lead to failure in changing the information security behaviour of consumers and employees. She has collaborated with government, law enforcement, and private sector organisations to assess national-level cybersecurity capacity and develop interventions to enhance resilience. She is a member of the National Risk Assessment (NRA) Behavioural Science Expert Group in the UK, working on the social and psychological impact of cyberattacks on members of the public. She is a member of the British Psychological Society and the British Counselling Society.

Philip Brining was awarded a BSc in hotel and catering management by the Polytechnic of North London in 1988. He read an MBA at Leeds Business School between 1991 and 1992 and launched a small food import and manufacturing business. In 1999 he went to work for Leeds United Football Club. In 2005 Phil set up Absolute Data, a consulting practice working with data, databases, and data protection/privacy. He founded Intelligent Sales, and then continued as a database consultant and data protection officer between 2010 and 2016. In 2015, Phil met Robin Hill and Andrew Mason and set up Data Protection People: a privacy and cybersecurity consultancy practice. In 2018, Phil was awarded a Master's degree in law (LLM) by the University of Northumbria. He became a Qualified Security Assessor (QSA) for the payment industry data security standard (PCI DSS) at around the same time. Phil lives in Great Ayton, North Yorkshire, and is married to Ann with whom he has three children. Away from work, his passions are dinghy sailing, camping, and brewing.

Rowenna Fielding is a freelance professional Privacy and Data Protection Consultant with over a decade of experience helping organisations stitch together law, technology, and humanity as best they can. An award-winning writer and educator, Rowenna has worked with charities, public sector organisations, and commercial businesses to improve data protection compliance and data ethics practices.

Cameron Broadbent started his career document writing within the legal sector. Looking for a new challenge he began working in cybersecurity. Now working for the cybersecurity awareness training company Bob's Business, he focuses on tackling the human side of cybersecurity. Cameron has produced a range of training content, articles, and more; all towards helping businesses to create and maintain a secure cybersecurity culture.

Melanie Oldham was awarded an OBE for Services to Cybersecurity in 2022 and has over 18 years of experience in cybersecurity. She is founder and CEO of Bob's Business, the cybersecurity awareness training company. Melanie has also created non-profit organisations to better integrate cybersecurity into society and the national curriculum in the UK. Melanie has spoken at various events around the world, helping to highlight the benefits that being secure online can bring to organisations and individuals alike.

Gary Hibberd is a Cybersecurity Consultant with over 27 years in the industry. Gary is an expert in information security, cybersecurity, and data protection, helping organisations large and small to make sense of their security processes and practices. Gary is also a published author, blogger, and speaker and co-owns a cyber security consultancy, Consultants Like Us, where they help businesses implement security frameworks such as ISO 27001, ISO 27701, and ISO 22301.

Mike Roberts has a wealth of experience in the field of e-signatures and secure email and has spent years helping businesses safeguard their electronic communications while streamlining the process for recipients. He has a proven track record of success and has assisted thousands of clients in achieving secure and efficient email communication.

Kim Page is a digital health entrepreneur, stemming from being the carer of a family member with a chronic condition. Based in Bedfordshire, UK, with over 20 years' experience that began in social care, her work has focused on improving the everyday lives of people in need, through strong systems and teams and through technology. Covering a decade of telehealth and telecare, leading system-wide strategy, right through to operational deployment, Kim's work focuses on the people and on the benefits that technology makes possible. With quality and accessibility in the spotlight, Kim has made the contribution to this publication after designing and launching Isosconnect, a platform for therapists and counsellors across disciplines to make online working safer and more effective for everyone.

Rory Lees-Oakes is a UK-based counselling tutor, trainer, therapist, and supervisor. He has been practising as a counsellor since 2003 and is a registered member of the National Counselling and Psychotherapy Society. Lees-Oakes has worked as a trainer and lecturer in counselling and psychotherapy at various colleges in the UK, including Tameside College, Warrington Collegiate, and various private training providers. In 2015, he was awarded a Silver Plato Award for outstanding use of technology education. He is the co-founder and academic director of Counsellor Tutor Ltd, an organisation that provides resources and training for counsellors and psychotherapists. He is also the co-host of the popular Counselling Tutor Podcast.

Elizabeth Milovidov is a lawyer from California, a law professor in Paris, France, and a former Digital Safety Consultant in Europe. Using her European/American focus on Internet, technology, and social media issues, she researches solutions to empower parents to guide their children in the digital age. Currently, she is the Global Digital Child Safety Lead supporting The LEGO Group as a trusted leader in implementing and promoting digital child safety, wellbeing, and citizenship in parallel with responsible digital engagement with children. She is the founder of DigitalParentingCoach.com, a website and community with resources for parents. Previous consulting projects included the Council of Europe (Children's Rights and Education departments), Microsoft (Digital Safety) and e-Enfance (Child Online Protection). She is an international speaker on digital parenting and safety and her work has been featured in WSJ, BBC, France 24, FOSI, Internet Matters, and other media outlets and organisations focused on child online safety.

Introduction

Why the book is needed

Catherine Knibbs

Why this book is needed

If you are reading this and work with 'clients' or 'patients' then it's likely you are within the scope of the health industry writ large, and you may have a specific social, psychological, or even emotional angle to your work. If you work directly with human bodies, such as chiropractors, massage therapists, or acupuncturists, then you most certainly fit within the health industry and follow the thinking and approaches offered in this book.

Some of the chapters address the profession of counselling and psychotherapy directly, but this is not to say the chapter, idea, or discussion should be skipped over or ignored, as many of the issues that practitioners face in training, further education, placements, private practice, associate work (self-employed), or within some types of organisations are relevant. Where you read what is written for the talking therapies these are not necessarily distinct from your work and role, so please make your way through all of the chapters. Also, the contributors are experts in their field – and not necessarily a practitioner within the health industries – and so this book has been created with many overarching principles and edits to reflect this.

Gaps, what gaps?

Many a conversation has been had within the industry of cybersecurity, data protection, and information governance revealing a deficit of knowledge across the board for many professions. This is something that I, Catherine, have been hearing about at many conferences (at one of which Gary and I met) over many years, and I have found it to be a topic, discipline, and approach that confuses many people in the health industry, as the legislation and policies in place speak to a 'generic population of professions' rather than those who hold and work with what I have always referred to as *sacrosanct* data. In this book, we will use this term throughout to denote people who attend sessions within the health industry (specifically counsellors, psychotherapists, and psychologists) because the work of this profession is the most profound space in which the following types of information are shared: any services delivered (such as therapy,

DOI: 10.4324/9781003364184-1

consultations, or audits) or criminal justice events, work-related conversations, secrets, wishes, desires, confessions, trauma, abuse, childhood events, politics, opinions, third-person data, fantasies, fetishes, kinks or sexual behaviours, emotions, tears and joy. Not to mention the work carried out with children that includes schools, services, courts, and medical and insurance company communication. Notwithstanding this, children create data if they work with creative media. They can possibly be recorded using video and audio. They may also be in settings where data is moved from one location to another and where the practitioners are both a joint controller and processor, as will be explained further in the book. When working from home using your own broadband Internet service provider (ISP), as happened throughout the lockdown periods and continues today in hybrid models, other considerations must be taken into account about how data, especially data about children, are accessed and shared and, of course, what you are liable for in terms of insurance under your professional working agreement with your ISP and your liability insurance company. If you are confused, worried, or want to walk away, now is the time to stick around and read the book for your own peace of mind and to protect the people you work with.

Computers and the ethereal space of digital

Since the inception of the computer, we have been, as a species, either fraught with excitement and a desire to use, learn, and integrate this into our lives, as both Gary and I have been – or not. And if not, the word often used to describe those who do not feel like this, or who might consider this technology an alien life form, is 'technophobe'. We are writing here for the technophobes. We are going to hold your hand through the book and provide a guide, with some tips, to help you achieve best practices for data.

There have been times over the past 100 years or so that sci-fi writings have speculated that we are heading for dystopian spaces – see, for example, the books *1984* (Orwell, 1949) and *The Singularity is Near* (Kurzweil, 2005). Or for an artificial intelligence (AI) takeover (at the time of editing, ChatGPT was emerging and had just appeared in the public domain); or the end of the world, with fabricated companies like Skynet, because of 'computers taking over the world', as in the 1984 movie, *The Terminator*. See https://www.imdb.com/title/tt0088247/.

And yet, the world found itself in a time and space in 2020 where a viral disaster (COVID-19) took over the world's day-to-day movements and face-to-face practices changed. This is still somewhat the case to date, where this very technology came to be a 'saviour' for some, a solution to isolation, and a much-needed tool for services to clients, patients, and customers in order to continue the provision of crucial services.

Contingency plans

However not all technophobes had a contingency plan (discussed later in the book), nor was this ever part of their world thinking and perhaps was never discussed in training – why would it be? Many technophobes thought the world would continue with 'normal service'. Gary and I, however, work in a world where anything can and does happen with technology and so the idea of backup plans, even when teaching and presenting, are a ubiquitous part of our daily work. You can't rely on technology and, given the pandemic, you can always rely on biology and Mother Nature to scupper your plans.

And so the reliance on technology that you may have is about to be challenged, and, by the end of the book, your provision of services and use of technology will mean that you will have that contingency plan set up, in order that you can be ready for Murphy's Law (also known as 'Sod's law' in some colloquial settings within the United Kingdom): '*Anything that can go wrong will go wrong, and at the worst possible time*' (see Wikipedia, https://en.wikipedia.org/wiki/Murphy's_law).

Technology, data protection, and the move into the digital age

I want to take you back to the inventions of worldwide communications afforded by technology – to the time of the telephone, then email, and then the Internet. But not entirely back to the *invention* of the telephone per se, rather to the legislation that appeared in 1998 alongside the World Wide Web only a few years before the millennium. What was called Y2K in the world of technology, and brought fears of failure and doom to the masses. As it turned out, the technologists got this (almost) right and the computers carried on with no real problems. Data from 31 December at 11:59 pm 1999 were still there the moment after midnight. TVs and washing machines were also fine, as were other communication channels such as the telephones working on electronic signals.

Telephones, fax machines and CCTV all belong in this conversation and thinking too, as you will see, and this often catches practitioners by surprise when Gary and I have a discussion with them about data protection that falls outside of this book's remit (we could not possibly include all areas of technology without making it into a tome).

The Data Protection Act of 1998

Now I am not going to reference the Data Protection Act from 1998 in full, because the point of this book is to bring you, the reader, up to date with the newest legislation so you can work and think using those best practices and begin making every decision towards data protection a normative part of your work. I am going to ask a question or two, set out below, to help set the scene for this book and to give you a roadmap of where you are going and what you need to do in order to move from technophobe, and unconsciously or consciously incompetent, to unconsciously competent. You will be able to build a set of principles, which you will meet more than once in this book, and using confidentiality, integrity, availability, and privacy as the four pillars of data protection, you can make the changes needed to ensure you practise lawfully and safely (meaning keeping things safe, and not needing to wear a 'hazmat suit').

It may help you to write down your answers to these questions, making a mind map to see how everything is connected, overlaps, and requires your basic knowledge of each and all of these areas. This book will help you get more detailed knowledge and so this exercise is the one I often use in training to 'set the scene'. Then we will address the specific deficits of knowledge that exist in these areas and why.

Questions

- Do you and have you used email to contact your place of work about work and clients/patients/customers? (If you are an associate, agency worker, or on placement see below.)
- Does this include your work as an associate, agency worker, placement?
- Do you use computers in the place of your associate, agency, or placement work?
- Do you own a phone that can send and receive text messages?
- Do you own a work, agency, or placement phone/device?
- Do you own a phone that can receive voicemail?
- Do you own a smartphone?
- Does your smartphone or device connect to the Cloud for backing up the device's contents?
- Do you connect your smartphone to a computer (for personal or professional purposes)?
- During training did you record your sessions (audio/video)?
- Do you record sessions now you have qualified (audio/video)?
- Did you use a Dictaphone or camera (not on a device)?
- Do you contact other organisations about your work, client, or customer base (e.g. social care, court, employment assistance programmes, insurance companies, health services, schools, or employers)?
- Do you use computers at home to type, send, or store any of the above?
- Do you write notes in a book or on paper and transport them to and from any of home, office, agency, employment, associate, meetings, court, etc.?
- Do you use a landline to make calls with or for any of the above?
- Do you have external devices that plug into your computer or device (e.g. a USB, SD card, or hard drive)?
- Is your computer or device connected to the Internet through ISP, 3G, 4G or 5G, or Wi-Fi?
- Do you use public Wi-Fi (e.g. cafes, food emporiums, trains, etc.)?
- Do you use Wi-Fi in the spaces you are attending training (e.g. conferences, hotels)?
- Do you access Wi-Fi or data on your devices when out of the country (e.g. on holiday)?
- Does your place of employment use CCTV?
- Does your house have a CCTV/Internet-connected camera (e.g. Ring)?
- Do you have a voice-activated system in your house (e.g. Alexa, Apple, TV, Smart TV)?

- Do you use any of the following: social media, dating apps, online banking, shopping apps, or home essentials on your smartphone, tablet, or computer?
- Do you wear a smartwatch?
- Do you track your own health data or log in to gym systems or other services (e.g. Strava)?

Reflection and pause

As you read through the questions, is there a connection being made about all these different versions of communication that you may in principle know about, but may not be an engineer, technical magician, or Elon Musk, and may not have a PhD or blueprint expertise in?

Had you considered that many of these areas overlap? Mostly, I find when teaching that when I begin to associate these answers with the most popular central tenant, we find that the smartphone and computer sit central to this. And most of the readers of this book will have both – and might even be reading this on or via one of them.

And has your training included within its curriculum, or your membership body explained, signposted, or provided training in, or have you otherwise been given training in data protection, cybersecurity, and privacy as a module or as continuing professional development? And if not, why not?

The book is born out of frustration

Often the answer to the above questions and reflections is a resounding no, so the training idea was born in 2018 via a conversation I had with several professionals in this area. We decided at the time that it would probably be more effective to provide training and to give people a way to establish good hygiene around these topics as the topic *de jour*: the General Data Protection Regulation (EU) (GDPR)was on the mind of many people in the UK. As the people who worked with sacrosanct data suddenly realised, they needed to practise ethically and diligently with the information customers, patients, and clients provided to them. Gary and I thought the world of counselling, psychotherapy, and psychology would be 'chomping at the bit', as they say, to bite off our hands for training in this area, given the expertise of the people who helped create the company with which to do this. We were sadly mistaken, as the resounding answer was: 'We have done the test on the ICO website and we don't need to register so we don't need the training.'

We, the cyber- and technology-based professionals were flummoxed. Surely, given the recent flurry of inbox emails we were all receiving as citizens of the UK, inundated by email requests from utility companies, businesses, and anyone else who held our data, with prompts, opt-ins, or opt-outs – and overwhelmed with what needed to be done and what were we opting in or out of anyway? So why was this profession at the time seemingly not recognising the need to take on training in data protection, cybersecurity, and privacy law and legislation, given it is still to this day missing from many of the sectors' training at college to university level environments? And why does it tend to cover the GDPR only? Why was technology safety missing, given the discipline of cybersecurity in business?

Many sectors pointed to the ICO as a way to say: 'What you have to do is over there' and this resulted in a mishmash of understanding about what being 'GDPR-compliant' meant or means (by the way, there's no such thing as you will find in this book). And, as a society (not just the profession of talking therapies), we (businesses) looked to tick-box exercises, training by the uprising of ready-made experts (there were lots of these suddenly appearing on social media selling their wares), profiteers, and organisations that were aimed at providing the bare basics and that did not fully understand the landscape of marketing, communications, technology, and information security that underpins or overlaps into the larger business models and practices involving technology (where misuse and misunderstandings of these sectors can cause issues, as you will read about in Chapter 4 on privacy). Some of the sole traders, small businesses or associates and employees who work from home had remote logins, or remote desktops, file transfer protocol (FTP) access, and worked with the most sensitive categories of information. (Discussed throughout the book.) Gary was even ejected from a social media group for challenging this behaviour – the group, which was for therapists only, had allowed him access – but, after realising he was not a therapist, he was removed (and so was Catherine). Online behaviours and groups are considered later in this book, looking at why these can be places where data can be mined and breaches can occur.

The product

I (Catherine) have harassed professionals from the world of data protection, cybersecurity, information governance, and privacy to write this book because I have been nagging them for five years to help. They have given their time to do this and previously have spent many an hour trying to answer my questions as to why this topic is so avoided and misunderstood, and why it has resulted in my now begging them to provide the contents herein. The book now in your hands has been a culmination of over five years of sleepless nights, angry blogs (which I accept full accountability for and still to exist to date), rants with cybersecurity and privacy experts, pleas to membership bodies, and my resignation from a director position where this topic was side-lined. This training often 'terrifies' the attendees, judging by the feedback I receive. For example, 'This is the first time we have heard about this', 'It is terrifying to think our devices and computers can be accessed like this', 'I thought I was compliant', 'What do you mean, read the DPA 2018?', 'I wasn't told I had to do this' – and the most saddening to hear: 'Our membership bodies have failed us' and 'Why would someone (meaning a cybercriminal) attack me, I help people?'; or 'But that's complicated and I can't be ***/bothered!'. The driving force behind this book, after being called a sensationalist or scary or accused of 'making it up' is the question: *'What's the worst that could happen?'*

The answer

Given that I, Catherine, the author of this introduction, have been an activist, pain in the rear, squeaky wheel and advocate for the clients, patients, and customers who are still to date (2023) being failed for many reasons, I took it upon myself to re-recruit the other editor of this book, Gary (who, having been in the industry for over 30 years, has been a staunch ally since the outset and offered his services to membership bodies, for free, to help them understand their obligations). We came to an agreement that the book needed to be in the hands of lots of professionals, as many practitioners may have grown tired of Catherine Knibbs alone explaining (I think they would use another word here) the laws and legislation. And so this book contains the same advice that I have been (irritatingly) spreading to those who wish I would go away. However, this is from the expertise of many who have worked in this field for over 30 to 40 years.

It's not my law, it's the law. It's compounded here by a range of academics, experts by experience and employment and education. I have merely been a messenger with over 30 years of working in this space of technology, with the privilege of being a psychotherapist, researcher, and author in this area also.

I do hope the ride throughout the text is *not* terrifying – but illuminating and guiding.

Why this book is for all levels of practitioner

From student to member body, from private practitioner to training institutes: why this book offers the foundational principle for all levels and why we all must take responsibility. The government provides the law and legislation (DPA, 2018), which is written for the plumber, dentist, book-keeper, gardener, and *you.*

There is a website online dedicated to providing support, guidance, and sign-posting to the most vulnerable of our society. The website is aimed at talking therapies and is a charity aimed at protecting the public from those who serve them in this profession. However, if you visit this website, there is Google geolo-cation installed that monitors your IP address (the address your Internet service provider gives your Internet connection). Your ISP can and does monitor all the websites you visit, and within their terms and conditions may share with other services and businesses. Those businesses can market to you directly or they can keep that information for their own purposes. Moreover, the website I am refer-ring to also has 'ad-trackers', which are discussed in Chapter 4 (on privacy) in more detail. The website does not disclose to you the purposes of the Google location or ad-trackers anywhere on its pages.

The issue here is that a person in emotional distress may not be in a state to consent to the processing of their data, and could even, under extreme circum-stances, be assessed under the Mental Health Act (1983) as not being in a fit mental state to consent to this process either, depending upon the level of stress or distress. Why is this important to consider here? If we consider the large respon-sibility the organisation has to the public, then I wonder where they have procured the guidance for their online presence and who approved the geoloca-tion process and under what remit? Now whilst it is not illegal to track a person's location, if you explicitly state the reason for needing this information, then we can see that there has very likely been a design flaw or reason for needing this information. However, the data protection laws are clear in explaining that you must inform people about what you are doing with their data, why, how long for, and what their rights are in relation to this. Given the website advises members to regularly remove cookies from their own computers, there is an inconsistency in the advice and guidance currently in place.

It became apparent through conversations with some of the contributors to this book, that current guidelines are what the author calls rounded shoulder policies, signposting practitioners to other sites to 'Do your own research', which of course is not illegal, nor as such classed as bad practice, however, these organisations are generally there to guide the students in training, the trainers who train them, and the practitioners when qualified in the 'best practice' – to prevent harm to the people they work with. When discussing the chapters with the authors in this book it was a general conversation that perhaps these bodies don't know what they need to advise their members, given that they are not in the large commercial or cor-porate sectors (such as banking, where large sums of money need to be protected, or insurance, or tightly controlled medical settings) where systems are created to protect customers.

And so, exposure to the issues of cybersecurity, information governance, privacy, and data protection has only just become the lexicon reaching the heads of the tables for the professions being spoken to in this book. In the space of online harm conversations at the time of writing, via the Online Safety Bill heading through parliament and the process of ratification (at the time of writing), I, Catherine, have already challenged the harms caused by professionals using technology without this backbone of foundational knowledge.

Apple watches and apps

A further issue to contemplate is the use of and recommendations for apps, gad-gets, and technology in practitioners' settings that are not understood in terms of data capture, use, or display settings. For example, many people own smart-watches, such as Apple watches. What would happen if the display showed the name and private message (e.g. a text) from a client, customer, or patient if the practitioner was wearing this device in close proximity to their client, patient, or customer? And the direct challenge to professionals in online spaces about these apps being used for surveillance, grooming, or data capture and mining that Catherine has made, is rejected, sneered at, or misunderstood – with answers like 'That *can't* be true', 'That's rubbish!', or 'You're being sensationalist' echoing through the comments. If recommendations are given to children and adults to use 'apps' that the practitioner is not well versed in themselves, or if these apps do not appear on a website such as Orcha (where these apps are rated, recommended, and scored on the measures of privacy and data protection), there is a real risk of data mining or of privacy issues; or, in the case of exploitative criminals, children being contacted for nefarious purposes. For example, what about apps that mine children's data or were created by predators and perpetrators of crimes against children? Yes, this really happens. (Please see Catherine's other writings, both on her website and in her books, about issues like this, because this is a very real risk for children.[1])

This book addresses the reduction in harm we all need to strive for and can be seen as a complement to and a 'manual' for many of the membership bodies, who often omit to guide, educate about the law, and provide training during training for the most sacrosanct form of data that exist (data entrusted to a professional by someone in distress). The contributors here all have that thinking within their writings, and so this book can be considered a guide in *how to reduce harm*, providing practitioners with guidance and education and, in doing so, reducing the likelihood of someone taking their own life, should the practitioner fail to protect that data.

Gratitude

I would like to thank the contributors of this book, all of whom are experts in the professional fields of cybersecurity, data protection, law, privacy rights, and education. Thank you to those who have worked with me for so long and understood my approach to getting this book into the hands of those who guard and protect people in so many ways. This book is a wonderful culmination of chapters that are written for practitioners and that will guide and help and ultimately may save a life. Thank you.

Note

1 Catherine Knibbs' books and blogs available via www.childrenandtech.co.uk.

References

Data Protection Act (1998). https://www.legislation.gov.uk/ukpga/2018/12/contents/enacted.

Data Protection Act (2018) https://www.legislation.gov.uk/ukpga/2018/12/contents/enacted.

General Data Protection Regulation (2018) https://gdpr-info.eu.

Kurzweil, R. (2005). *The Singularity Is Near: When Humans Transcend Biology*. Viking

Mental Health Act (1983) https://www.legislation.gov.uk/ukpga/1983/20/contents.

Murphy's Law. https://en.wikipedia.org/wiki/Murphy's_law.

Orcha Health (n.d.) https://orchahealth.com.

Orwell, G. (1949, republished 2008). *1984*. Penguin, in association with Martin Secker & Warburg.

The Terminator (1984). https://www.imdb.com/title/tt0088247.

1 Cyberethics, philosophy, and ethics

Catherine Knibbs

Metaphilosophy, metaphysics, and cyberethics

Nomenclature seems to be the art of confusing people with language about a particular topic, and so, like most academic writings, this chapter will be no different in describing the issue faced today by practitioners in their existence around and the use of technology to provide services to clients or patients.

We live in a world that is ubiquitous with technology and has been for many years. One of the complexities of this chapter is to discuss, without jargon (where possible), the need to understand how this technology works with, for and against us when we operate in the sector of mental health where this technology is ever-present. Much of the last decade has been focused on the use cases of this technology and how to provide services in a manner that replicates the real world. Sadly, it took a worldwide pandemic to create an integration of this technology into those spaces for the technologically avoidant or resistant practitioners. Many have done so without a foundation for good and ethical practice and the author posits that many people may well have been harmed by this process, in respect of data mining, breaches of data protection laws, surveillance capitalistic manoeuvres by 'big tech' and the impact of this may not be truly recognised for decades.

This chapter exists within this book to emphasise the beginnings of conversations that have been, in the author's professional opinion, sadly missing from this sector for many years, as the world of technology, information, data governance, and cyber protection when using technology has been surreptitiously missed, omitted and is lacking in good guidance (to date) for the sectors that hold the most sacrosanct information in the professions that exist in the world.

Where else are secrets, wishes, desires, trauma, abuse, war, atrocities, and childhood distress kept but in the hands of those who once listened in real-world offices and clinics, to only now be kept in a permanent format accessible by bad actors when not protected? This format is liable to intrusion, breaches, exposure, corruption, and decay by practitioners who may not be versed in knowing how to protect and keep this safe.

The why? Well, that is the remit of this book. This chapter will address the ethical landscape and propose what changes need to take place, what needs to be included going forward, and what standards need to be created to protect the public now, in the past, and in the future.

DOI: 10.4324/9781003364184-2

Why do we need an ethical paradigm for technology?

Briefly, for the reader, beginning with some metaphysical and philosophical concepts to highlight where the deficits in this space may be, why we need to consider these stances and approaches to our use of technology and why we are summarily actors, users, creators, and responsible parties to this technology, where it appears in our practice and daily lives, and why do these two terrains overlap, and why do we need to consider our use of technology and how this can create risk for the patients and clients we work with (as well as for us as individuals).

Computer ethics. This was described in 1985 as:

> an analysis of the nature and social impact of computer technology and the corresponding formulation and justification of policies for the ethical use of such technology.
>
> (Moor, 1985, p. 266)

This quote stood out as the author respectfully agrees that this is still true today – and this was written nearly 40 years ago from the time of writing. This does not refer to the 'acceptable use policies' about social media but *the ethical policies* for use of such technology with clients or patients, beyond what is currently available. Moor continues: 'Often, no policies for conduct in these situations exist or existing policies seem inadequate' (1985, p. 266).

And so, the first question for the readers of this book right here at the outset is: Where do you find or follow such policies and are there any in your profession? Did you even know there was such a thing? Do you have your own policies other than 'acceptable use' guides or data protection or privacy polices?

And, so we move to another way to see the issues we face as practitioners and the essence of guidance for us 'using' technology to support our practices.

Cyberethics is suggested to be: 'a branch of applied ethics that examines moral, legal, and social issues at the intersection of computer/information and communication technologies' (Tavani, 2013; Spinello, 2017, 2021).

Isn't this 'just' ethics writ large?

Now some readers may be thinking that these ethics are 'just the same as the real-world ethics we face'. Floridi (1999) suggests the idea that computer ethics is more macro than micro, with, for example, macro being an overarching philosophy and micro being specific to industry. He argues there is a particular distinction for computer ethics that is not replicable in the real world, often conceived of as magical environments, but has real-world consequences making it more than an industry form of ethics. For example, you have probably heard people say it's the technology that is at fault, for example, it 'glitched'. Floridi called these dismissive reports of computer errors and not the user. This highlights the lack of understanding of these reports as to why a computer glitched or didn't run the program when, at the time of writing, computers are not sentient beings that can make choices about what they are instructed to 'do'. The removal of oneself from responsibility in this way is why the author is suggesting that these approaches *must* be included in the spaces of mental health and digital technologies.

Whilst these concepts so far encompass the idea that this is about the issues that you are facing as a 'user' of this technology, you are also a practitioner who is controlling and processing the data that belongs to your client or patient and as such have a responsibility to look after, protect, and guard that data in the space of a digital landscape and remit. And you will need the skills and thinking of cyberethics as well as the understanding to do this competently.

Whilst the disciplines of cyberethics and computer ethics do not necessarily form the contents of this book as a specific topic matter, nevertheless, it is imperative that, under the umbrella of cyberethics, I (the author) include your professional work here to include the issues of information security, privacy, and data protection.

This book is not large enough to take you through the complexities of cyberethics, how the Internet 'works', or why indeed you are now seeing this word, for what may be the first time in relation to being a practitioner in the field of psychology, psychotherapy, counselling, or other health-related professions such as social or youth work, safeguarding, or even disciplines such as chiropractic, aromatherapy, or other types of body therapies.

Therefore, this chapter is seated at the start of the book to create a space for you to think in an ethical and pragmatic way, and to introduce you to the chapters that follow as all of them form a manual of sorts, for your profession, so you can practice within the law, do so as safely and securely as possible, and have the least amount of anxiety related to this discipline. Safe and secure are not typically how talking therapies think of these words as they are specific to the digital landscape within this book and so your lexicon is likely to broaden and in doing so consider these words in relation to technology rather than the alliance of psychological safety, trauma safety, body safety, and so on.

What *is* technology and *why* cyberethics?

Whether you use a digital telephone (the old-fashioned one that plugs into the wall and may have a voicemail system attached to it), a smartphone, or even a computer to communicate with your patients and clients, there is a responsibility for you to know what it is that occurs in the storage, use, and transmission of that data, what your part in the process is, and what you need to consider in that ethical framework. You don't need to be a technical genius or a programmer or understand Boolean logic and binary code.

Throughout this chapter and indeed the rest of the book, the contributors are seated in a position that mirrors Spinello, (2017; 2021) with the following quote:

> We implicitly embrace the philosophy of technological realism, which sees technology as a powerful agent for change and forward progress in society. But, unlike more utopian views, this position does not ignore the dangers and

deterministic tendencies of technology along with its potential to cause harm and undermine basic human rights and values.

(p. xi, Preface, 2017)

The use of technology requires us to know what these dangers could be, how these deterministic spaces can create social injustice issues and discrimination, and how the technology can 'spy' on those people you are using the technology *with*.

Ethics can often be a topic that, when synced up with the idea of 'cyber' or digital, results in eye-rolls of magnitude that a teenager might be jealous of. These topics are fraught with some avoidance, neglect, and even hatred of such. They are profoundly entrenched in the speculative feelings and thinking of mights and coulds and the philosophy of 'it will never happen to me'. This thinking about cyberethics is not reserved for the professions of psychology, counselling, and sole traders in the field of mental health alone. This is indeed why the fields of information security, cybersecurity, data protection, and privacy exist, and have done since the use of the computer in work and home settings became the norm. They are going to continue to do so for as long as digital technology forms part of the working world.

Do I have to?

This avoidance of the topics named above is apparent in the uptake of courses, books, and seminars that exist in the mental health and wellbeing fields with wording in the titles being cyberethics, cybersecurity, data protection, or privacy, and in how few people want to attend these events versus those that are fluffy and nice like 'learn how to paint' or 'buzzword bingo' – popular and easy to navigate sources of learning, continuing professional education, or webinars. The evidence for this? Over five years of this author providing such courses and conversations with large and small organisations and membership bodies who don't know what they don't know, and don't know what they need to provide for their members in order that they can practise safely, ethically, and lawfully using digital technologies. This is echoed in the fields of online safety, online harm, and, outside of the National Health Service, as to what sole traders, students on placement, training institutes, and even perhaps colleges need to know about best practices when it comes to the risks and dangers of using technology and how you can protect yourself, your patients, and your clients. And it's been missing since 1996, 1998 and 2018 (these years are important throughout the book).

Moreover, those smaller organisations have on occasion decided to negate their duties in favour of 'it's too complicated', 'requires me to read a lot of policies', or require them to rewrite some of their own material. In doing so, this book idea was born out of frustration and a need to challenge the ethics of what felt like a teenager's response to being asked to tidy their room.

Cyberethics, or more accurately ethics, requires you to think for yourself, and to consider what is right and 'proper', in order to protect the rights and freedoms offered to those people, those humans that you work with, people that the cyber aspect is directed to when using technology. It's not easy to be thinking about the risks and dangers of digital technology if you don't know what they are, and if you think that you will not be affected by them under the cognitive bias of cyber-criminals avoiding targeting you because you care for other people (and are therefore altruistic, kind, and 'nice'), are only small as a business, or are even a student in training. If you don't know about how digital technology works, then why would this be a part of your thinking? After all, as the author regularly states in training: police are taught how to police, teachers to teach, and doctors how to save lives. You didn't sign up to be a cyber expert or technological genius, you just want to help the person you are working with and provide a service using today's technology. The question most often posed at this point is: 'Well, what's the worst that can happen?' (See the chapters in this book to find out those answers.)

Training through to practice: From beginner to master craftsperson

In order to get to practitioner status at the end of your course, you have to learn the ropes, you are often taught what ethics are and your thinking towards this subject as you progress through the scenarios offered by tutors during your training. You must consider your own fallibility and biases, and where you might have errors of judgement, 'isms', and distortions in your thinking. The world of cyber-ethics is a whole new world of future thinking and potentials, and the chapter I refer you to as the reader is the introduction to why this book is needed in the first place, because cyberethics is not something often taught in the early phases of practitioner training. It's the aspect of police are taught to 'police' and uphold the law, teachers are taught to 'teach the curriculum', and you were taught to 'work with people' through talking, touch, or interventions, often in the here and now, and this may well be an issue in the future when it comes to digital data and what that means for you as a professional.

Let's start with what you are taught

If you are a professional reading this and work with 'clients' or 'patients' then it's likely you are within the scope of the health industry writ large and, for example, may have a social, psychological, or even emotional angle to your work. If you work directly with human bodies, such as chiropractors, massage therapists, or acupuncturists, then you most certainly fit within the health industry and follow the thinking and approaches offered in this book.

When you sign up to take your course you could be at the level of attending your local college for a Level 2, 3 or 4 Certificate or Diploma, you could be doing a top-up degree or a degree without research at be at Level 5, or you could be taking the longer courses providing you with a level of 6, 7, or heading into the world of Level 8, in which case you are likely to be conducting research. If you conduct research as part of your training you will undoubtedly come across ethics as a mandatory part of how to carry out research and with that, you will learn the terminology that will feel familiar as you read this chapter. However, if you have never had to consider the issues around words like informed consent (not to be confused with the data protection language here), beneficence, maleficence, extortion, exploitation, or researcher bias, then this chapter is going to address new language for you. These words are easy enough to research so they will not be explained in depth, and they will be used as and when necessary. In the words of many investors, DYOR (do your own research) in order that you can follow along.

Primum non-nocere: First do no harm

At the outset of your training, you begin with the approach of considering who you serve professionally and your responsibility to them. In the health industry and occupations when and where this is medically orientated there is a legend, myth, and actuality of the Hippocratic oath, often regurgitated as '*first, do no harm*' (which is said to appear in Hippocrates' work called '*Of the Epidemics*' (http://classics.mit.edu/Hippocrates/epidemics.1.i.html) and not his strict instructions to practitioners worldwide). However, taking this approach, the 'doing of no harm' implies that the harm must be understood by the practitioner. For example, a doctor or paramedic in training is educated about harm and the prospect of saving lives as the primary outcome in the face of this dilemma. An example this could be the extreme case of needing to amputate a limb to save a life, and I suspect not many of us would argue this point. (Unless you are partial to courtrooms and litigation processes, or because you feel you would have made better decisions than the paramedics or doctors did at the moment of incision. And who among us is ever in this life-or-death decision-making process with the data we process?)

But what about your role as someone using technology who isn't in crisis mode and requires a rushed response to using technology (aside from March 2020), when controlling, manipulating, and processing the data, information, and details that belong to someone else? Effectively their sensitive health data. How do you 'do no harm' if you don't know how those harms can occur?

Training and the route to ethical practice in practice

The discipline under which you are training, for example, the humanities such as social work, psychology, counselling, or perhaps youth work, approaches ethics in a particular way when it comes to your learning, as it is often applied to your actual professional role and not the administrative task or, as posited early on in this chapter, cyberethics or computer ethics. The coursed is designed to lead you to be able to practise your profession and profess your qualifications to highlight your professionalism to the public. This likely means that when you sign up for your course there is a carrot on the end of the stick in terms of accreditation, registration, or approved qualifications that you can achieve either at the end of the course or the end of your professional training journey. And the subsidiary of this is likely to be a membership body or service that you pay to advertise those credentials to the public to assure them you're suitably qualified. Telling the public you are versed in ethical assumptions and practice is often not required, and the public will assume that you are indeed an ethical practitioner based on your qualifications.

The public can place their trust in these systems because the membership bodies make this clear through regulatory bodies, declare this through their visibility in the public domain, and display this on their website and in their communications, and some also have an approved registration process as part of the membership body (for example, the Professional Standards Authority for health and social care (PSA) (https://www.professionalstandards.org.uk/home) who oversee the registers that each membership body has. Or the Health and Care Professionals Council (HCPC) (https://www.hcpc-uk.org/), which has some ethical frameworks and guidance available on its website available for the public to see as well. The membership bodies can be large associations, like the British Psychological Society (BPS) (which has a cyberpsychology division too) (https://www.bps.org.uk/), or smaller associations that oversee specific approaches to health and wellbeing. In the space of talking therapies, the main membership bodies are: the United Kingdom Council for Psychotherapy (https://www.psychotherapy.org.uk/), the National Counselling Society (https://nationalcounsellingsociety.org/), the British Association for Counselling and Psychotherapy (https://www.bacp.co.uk/), and the British Psychoanalytic Society (https://psychoanalysis.org.uk/). There are also membership bodies for child-based services such as British Association for Play Therapists (https://www.bapt.info/), Play Therapy UK (https://playtherapy.org.uk/), and the British Association for Art Therapy (https://baat.org/) – and so many more (it is said there are approximately 250-plus associations, approaches, and disciplines so these are not all listed here). And, of course, there are all the other disciplines and approaches in the health and wellbeing fields.

So where is the overarching cyberethics, or indeed one-stop-shop and coherent model that all these professional roles can adhere to or follow with regard to technology use, protection of information, and data protection? Where are the standard operating procedures akin to those you would find for engineering for example? You guessed it. We are still developing some of these and, to date, the author cannot find on any one of these member bodies or authorities' websites a set of cyberethics for you to follow as a practitioner or a coherent document with all of the above contained in one place to guide you lawfully in your practice. There are some good practice guides (some pointing to online work, which is reasonable) and ethical guidelines, but there are way too many scattered links and clicks and documents on many different pages, with some of these giving 404 notifications (broken webpages); and lots of the advice to date is contradictory, depending upon who has written it and what role they have in the membership bodies. This is confusing and unhelpful to the practitioner and the public.

The synthesis of technology and ethics is omitted. And the most worrying part for many of the authors in this book is that the guidelines and best practices don't necessarily communicate that data protection is a law, not an option, and that legislation can see you fined or prevented from working by removing your right to control or process data should that be the outcome (very unlikely for a first-time offence, but nonetheless a cautionary note).

For example, on the HCPC website, there are ethical guidelines for practice and record-keeping, which tell you to keep accurate records and to protect them from discovery, loss, and destruction, and that the resources you need are elsewhere on the sites of organisations such as the Information Commissioners Office (ICO). They even have guidance on the use of social media in respect of your patients or clients seeing what you post, yet discussions about the messenger systems, business profiles, or security of these systems are missing. On the PSA site, there is no ethical framework, as this is not what they do: they oversee membership bodies' registers. If you visit the BPS and search for their policies and guidelines, you will find the Practice Guidelines dated August 2017 available for access. BPS has updated most of its website in recent months (and indeed over the last year or so, and it has a link for frequently asked questions about website content that you cannot find (https://www.bps.org.uk/faqs/what-can-i-do-if-i-cant-find-what-im-looking-website)), however, some of the hyperlinks in the 2017 document do not work either.

However, you can see here that the author does not attack this document as being dated before 2018 as some of the advice is still helpful and relevant, but in a complementary approach quotes directly from this guide are provided from Section 7:

7.1 Information Governance

Psychologists should follow local and national guidance and statutory responsibilities regarding management of data. Psychologists should make, keep and disclose information in records only in accordance with national policy and legislation, and the policies and procedures of the organisation(s) they are employed by/working in collaboration with.

(p. 55)

This paragraph still rings true to date and so is in line with current legislation. Sadly, it does not contain information in detail about the Data Protection Act 1998 (see https://www.legislation.gov.uk/ukpga/1998/29/contents) aside from the mention in the confidentiality and safeguarding section (and as part of the current legislation appendix), nor can it mention the Data Protection Act 2018, as the document is prior to that date. There are, however, updated articles on the BPS site answering some questions about General Data Protection Regulation (GPDR) and technology (you have to search for them in resources). *Section 2.2* specifically addresses working in a digital age and gives some advice about security measures for practitioners, signposting for the keeping of these. It recommends:

Digital media continues to advance in terms of choice and functionality. It is becoming increasingly common for psychologists in particular when working with clients to make use of the internet and/audio-visual technology. These technologies require the psychologist to ensure that the network used is as secure as reasonably possible and, as far as is feasible, assures privacy to their clients.

It also points to the processes of standards and security measures when using technology (valid at the time), advising:

> Some employers may have their own rules about which media are acceptable to use. The USA has the Health Insurance Portability and Accountability Act (HIPAA) which sets standards for security for electronic data. There is no such provision in the UK to date, and so psychologists must satisfy themselves that any media used to communicate personal data is secure. This is a rapidly changing area and so technology-specific guidance has not been provided in this document. There can be no guarantee of security when using the internet, and voice over internet protocol (VOIP) services such as 'Skype' or 'FaceTime' are no different, as they use the same data infrastructure as the rest of the internet. Most, if not all, VOIP systems encrypt the voice into waveforms during digital transit across the internet, and it would be impossible to eavesdrop on these data packets in real time. However, the information is potentially vulnerable to eavesdropping/compromise before encryption by the speaker's system, and after decryption by the listener's system. This will depend upon the security measures in place for the end user's (speaker and listener) own networking infrastructures, be that a company, institution or home user. If an end user's computer has been compromised by any form of malware, then there will be a risk of eavesdropping, data theft and/or denial of service. The risk for eavesdropping on VOIP systems is no more or less than that of traditional analogue phone systems, and both would require specialist knowledge, equipment and software to be achieved. However, it is recommended that only fit-for-purpose VOIP systems are used, and that public networks, such as Social Media sites, are avoided for VOIP communications.

Given that this document has been in circulation since 2017, the author was surprised to find that many of the other membership bodies mentioned above did not utilise or expand on this framework, given the changes in 2018 to the Data Protection Act, the introduction of The General Data Protection Regulation (2018) (https://gdpr-info.eu/) as an aspect of the Act and also where the inclusion of other legislation was, or why this was omitted given many practitioners who are sole traders utilise email, marketing, social media, and other forms of contact with and through technology.

Moreover, the Data Protection Act 2018, and the case laws surrounding Max Schremms, namely *Schremms ii* (there is also *i* and allegedly soon to be *iii*) would highlight very quickly that practitioners based in the UK and EU as well as US-based platforms cannot guarantee the data remains within the EU, and therefore require the use of Standard Clause Certificates (SCC). Furthermore, in 2022 these were superseded by the International Transfer Data Act (ITDA), which governs how practitioners must inform their patients and clients about the use of these platforms in their privacy policy, detailing the risk involved (https://ico.org.uk/for-organisations/guide-to-data-protection/guide-to-the-general-data-protection-regulation-gdpr/international-data-transfer-agreement-and-guidance/) The chapters that follow address these issues in greater detail and so the rest of this chapter will address the ethical issues of concern.

Ethical considerations

The rest of this chapter is going to bring some questions that are applicable to both practitioners and training bodies about what is required of the user, processor, and controllers of data, and what may need to be in data protection policies, training standards, and considerations about the technology that is outside of awareness and production in 2023. Many of these questions are taken from a white paper (in press) regarding the International Coalition of Mental Health and Virtual Reality (MHVR) that the author has written, and which are applicable to all forms of technology being used in today's society. Two further additions here the disciplines of neuro rights (find out more here https://neurorightsfoundation. org/) and ethics, which are about the collection of data that is biometric, related to health (wearables), emotions, brain wave patterns and implants that can detect real-time feedback. Given the recent overturn of *Roe versus Wade (1973)* in the United States (https://supreme.justia.com/cases/federal/us/410/113/), tracking data that is of this nature can expose practitioners to many issues; this practice is likely to expand beyond the United States – for example, in the cases of murder, homicide, assault, and abuse – and practitioners may need to present this kind of evidence in criminal justice systems and cases if we do not take action on this in the coming years. What constitutes good practice versus confidentiality, versus what can be subpoenaed?

Leaving this huge dilemma behind here in this chapter, the author is moving the reader to questions about technology in use today and where the ethical dilemmas are in respect of cybersecurity, data protection, and privacy laws before moving to these chapters in more detail. The following passages are taken from the above-mentioned white paper (in press) regarding virtual reality (VR). (There may be some repetition of the above conversations, and the reader is asked to bear with this for now.)

White paper (in Press)

Given the broad range of uses for technology, communication via such technologies, and the emerging uses of augmented reality- and virtual reality-based interventions in health-related services such as counselling and psychotherapy through to in-house hospital and hospice delivery, it was deemed that, for the white paper written about VR, consideration would be given to the ethical frameworks surrounding these spaces, places, and services. In doing this it became apparent that whilst many health-related services have ethical frameworks for the professions as a whole, or for the delivery of services, there is a deficit of frameworks surrounding *the uses of data therein* and how to adequately use, protect, and share data with others abiding by the laws of the Data Protection Act (2018) and the GDPR (2018).

This is highly likely to be due to the exponential speed of technology in settings of mental health and wellbeing as a whole and, as such, the professional bodies that oversee the ethics, due diligence, and health and safety aspects are behind in both the discussions and the implementation of ethical frameworks around the use of this equipment. This may, in part be attributable to the lack of understanding of how the technology works or communicates with other systems online, 'in the cloud', or via platforms, how this aspect complicates the rights of users, and how it can be used or misused by both the practitioner or the providers. Other speculative reasons for this delay are not discussed in this chapter. However, this can be briefly seen to be further complicated by the frameworks of how newer technologies such as video, VR, and immersive spaces and domains span into other disciplines, such as privacy rights and freedoms, data protection, neuro rights, and biometric data creating an expanding field of what will need to be professional training, guides, websites, and standards. This approach would require multidisciplinary conversations about these areas and discussion about the best way to create, design, and incorporate the ethical frameworks needed.

If, however, we can, through the white paper here and in extension, create direct communication with legislative bodies and technology providers (or big tech), it could lead to the exemplar of how to create a set of ethical assumptions about the use of technology – in this case, VR for use in clinical settings. Given that this white paper is likely to extend into health settings outside counselling and psychotherapy, and may well include the sectors of wellbeing, crisis support, criminal justice, social care, and education, this illuminates the issue of how such an ethical framework can be created, communicated, and implemented if there is not a universal body of collaboration between professions that may find themselves using the equipment. For example, in education, youth and outreach work settings, this equipment is also used, and again is without a framework for the ethical considerations of how the equipment and apps and programs on it are used as well.

Creating a universal ethical framework is both a theoretical and pragmatic issue that is being highlighted here in the white paper. To consider this issue, the following information is being posited for the thoughtful processes that surround each issue, and whilst there are no clear-cut answers at this stage, it is hoped this will create the discussions needed in the many sectors and professions that will use such equipment now and in the future. To do this, case examples will be given to highlight the ethical, practical, and legal aspects that will be required to create a framework that can transition many disciplines, professions, and interventions or uses. To date there is a broad-brush approach of considerations – for example, a report looking at the growing value of extended reality (XR) (immersive technology) in the UK has a short reflection on the challenges faced when using this technology as well as the values and benefits. It is clear from the report that many cases have been cited of the benefits of this technology, however, it is unclear where any of the studies followed an ethical framework or, indeed, whom this framework is written by, or where it exists. This further highlights the need for professional or member bodies to create such a framework, as currently there are guidelines, laws, and standards for the area of data protection and privacy as highlighted by the XRSI [Extended Reality Safety Intelligence] Privacy Framework (2020) and the expanding use of XR in health care (2022).

The white paper (in press) also has some case use examples and one that is applicable to this book and the contents is provided here for the reader.

Use of online spaces

E-Safety/Online Safety/Confidentiality

In some cases, programs and apps can be used remotely to meet with a client or patient in an environment where other users may be present. Protecting the patient's anonymity, confidentiality, and privacy is paramount and may not be possible in a shared VR environment. This paper suggests that communication (audio) may need to take place using a parallel system such as those that meet the GDPR and HIPPA compliance standards and keeping communication via the VR environment to a minimum (for example, turning off microphones on the headset) until there is an app that meets the data protection and confidentiality requirements mentioned. It is unknown whether some platforms could record discussions taking place between the practitioner and patient/client and therefore audio conversations will need to be protected. Practitioners should ensure the confidentiality of their sessions where they can take actions to protect this, until these apps and platforms can guarantee within their Terms & Conditions and privacy policies they are committed to and are following data protection, security, and privacy law and practice.

Post-session sign-ups to platforms and apps

The questions arising here may not necessarily be pertinent to the session taking place between professional and client as, post-meeting, the individual patient or client, who may have significant vulnerabilities (such as being a child or having educational difficulties), may sign into these spaces/platforms online, but not have received (or understood) protective education in online safety, or may have other vulnerabilities (relational), and so may be at significant risk of grooming or other forms of crimes being committed upon them. This raises the issue of children using online spaces, platforms, and apps that they have been introduced to without parental oversight or education from the practitioner about those very spaces being used. Moreover, if the practitioner is not present to guide and facilitate, or if the practitioner does not have an awareness of basic online safety skills and resources in order to provide children with valuable resources and safeguarding education, this could also result in children being at risk of online harms. Who will train the practitioner or patient or both in this aspect and how will this be regulated, overseen, or otherwise?

Data protection, privacy, and adequate training for practitioners

Use of equipment that is owned by a corporation with cloud facilities may result in the following types of issues.

In many cases, the current landscape of VR headsets belongs to organisations such as Meta, Sony, and HTC, requiring the user to create an account with them for the purposes for use of that equipment. In doing so, akin to digital health apps, the user would in most cases be the practitioner or clinical staff. However, if separate patient accounts are created in the system, then what measures are in place to keep that data confidential, safe, and out of reach of data-mining and surveillance practices? Where does a practitioner find the guidance to create a contract and user agreement with the patient about using these devices, and what data is collected by them in order to use the system; for example, some apps allow for 'multiple users' and, when doing so, are users required to submit sensitive categories of data such as date of birth? In this use case, does the platform then hold this data, or the app, or the practitioner, or is it all three? It is suggested here that the ethical guidelines incorporate information on reducing the collection of data about the practitioner's clients/patients, or that practitioners who create accounts on the systems reduce the likelihood of personal information being collected about the clients/patients. If practitioners are to use VR environments, how can they give their clients/patients with a robust understanding about what data will be collected about them by the platform, app, or tech company, and so provide an opportunity for informed consent before 'adding' the user or allowing them to use those systems? How is biometric data protected and what considerations need to be applied to an ethical framework here?

It is noted that the use of many of these VR technologies and the apps, systems, and platforms created are not intended for clinical use, and therefore most of the Terms & Conditions are ineffective for these situations. This creates difficulty for both the everyday user as well as the practitioner about how they protect their own rights and freedoms while being enabled to use the spaces freely, as well as the expectations of clinical use and the protection of people in those settings.

Moreover, if data is created by the user (for example, images, creative aspects such as avatars, and so on), which the program allows for retrieval and sharing, then that data will be collected by the program (including biomedical data). How is this protected? And what framework would oversee this in terms of a practitioner's responsibility and training in order to use these facilities, within or through the programs, and to be able to print, email, or capture this data securely and safely? How can the practitioner ensure the data is not hacked or tampered with and what training is required for such a requisite?

What could this data imply about a person's health? Whose responsibility is it to monitor that health data and whom can this be shared with, and how, and what procedures and guidance are in place for practitioners using this equipment and who need to be able to move data from device to shareable formats? How competent and tech-savvy are they?

Case uses may include practitioners who are not versed in some of the above issues and this could result in accidental data exposure, collection or breaches, misuse of programs, and lack of awareness of the side effects of such a breach, and may inadvertently create psychological and emotional injuries to the users through lack of knowledge about the issues raised. This brings to light where, how, and when a complaint can be brought and what would be the correct channel for doing so?

Insurance, complaints, and the responsibility of the practitioner

Lastly, ethical considerations for insurance, including cyber-insurance bring another layer of complexity to the framework, as this type of equipment or data is not necessarily included in policies for liability. Many insurance companies providing liability and practice complaints insurance do not cover cyber-related attacks or breaches where the practitioner failed to use what are called under the GDPR 'all technical and organisational measures' to protect such data. For example, if a practitioner failed to implement basic cybersecurity measures and protection on their devices, would they be covered in the event of an attack, breach, or misuse of technology as detailed above in some of the examples? Whether this would need separate insurance to cover the practitioner is unclear as the standards for the use of VR in mental health are also a grey area. Currently, one insurance service in the UK provides cyber-insurance for professionals discussed in this paper.

Further reading

Bostrum, N. (2014) *Superintelligence. Paths, Dangers, Strategies.* Oxford: Oxford University Press.

Bynum, T.W. (2008). Milestones in the history of information and computer ethics. The Handbook of Information and Computer Ethics. Hoboken, NJ: John Wiley & Sons. 25–48.

Gert, B. (1999). Common morality and computing. *Ethics and Information Technology, 1*(1), 53–60.

Goodman, K.W. (1998). Bioethics and health informatics: An introduction. *Biomed Ethics, 4*(2), 40–47.

Johnson, D.G. (1985). *Computer Ethics.* Hoboken, NJ: Prentice Hall.

Moor, J.H. (2001). The future of computer ethics: You ain't seen nothin' yet! *Ethics and Information Technology, 3*(2), 89–91.

Tavani, H.T. (2003). Ethics and technology: Ethical issues in an age of information and communication technology. *ACM SIGCAS Computers and Society, 33*(3).

Tavani, H.T. (2004). Genomic research and data-mining technology: Implications for personal privacy and informed consent. *Ethics and Information Technology, 6*(1), 15–28.

Tavani, H.T. (2006). *Ethics at the Intersection of Computing and Genomics.* London: Jones and Bartlett.

References

Data Protection Act (1998) https://www.legislation.gov.uk/ukpga/1998/29/contents.

Data Protection Act Legislation (2018) https://www.legislation.gov.uk/ukpga/2018/12/contents/enacted.

Floridi, L. (1999). Information ethics: On the philosophical foundation of computer ethics. *Ethics and Information Technology, 1*(1), 33–52.

GDPR (2018) https://gdpr-info.eu.

HIPAA (n.d.) https://www.hhs.gov/hipaa/index.html.

Moor, J.H. (1985). What is computer ethics?. *Metaphilosophy, 16*(4), 266–275.

Tavani, H.T. (2013). Cyberethics. In Runehov, A.L.C., Oviedo, L. (Eds), *Encyclopedia of Sciences and Religions.* Springer, Dordrecht.

Spinello, R. (2017). *Cyberethics: Morality and Law in Cyberspace.* 6th Edition. Burlington, MA: Jones & Bartlett Learning.

Spinello, R. (2021). *Cyberethics: Morality and Law in Cyberspace.* 7th Edition. Burlington, MA: Jones & Bartlett Learning.

Website references

https://baat.org/

http://classics.mit.edu/Hippocrates/epidemics.1.i.html

https://ico.org.uk/for-organisations/guide-to-data-protection/guide-to-the-general-data-protection-regulation-gdpr/international-data-transfer-agreement-and-guidance/

https://nationalcounsellingsociety.org/

https://neurorightsfoundation.org/

https://playtherapy.org.uk/

https://psychoanalysis.org.uk/

https://www.bacp.co.uk/

https://www.bapt.info/

https://www.bps.org.uk/

https://www.bps.org.uk/faqs/what-can-i-do-if-i-cant-find-what-im-looking-website

https://www.bps.org.uk/guideline/general-data-protection-regulation-gdpr-faqs

https://www.hcpc-uk.org/

https://www.hhs.gov/hipaa/index.html

https://www.professionalstandards.org.uk/home/

https://www.psychotherapy.org.uk/

Roe vs Wade (1973). https://supreme.justia.com/cases/federal/us/410/113/.

XR Health UK (2022). The growing value of XR in health care. Accessed online at https://www.xrhealthuk.org/the-growing-value-of-xr-in-healthcare.

The XRSI Privacy Framework Version 1.0 (2020). https://xrsi.org/publication/the-xrsi-privacy-framework.

2 A clinician's guide to cybersecurity and data protection

How to ensure client confidentiality?

Maria Bada

1 Introduction

Current developments in electronic healthcare technology have led to exponential improvements in clinical outcomes and have transformed care delivery. This means that not only services but also data have now moved online in most parts of the world. Also, electronic health records (EHRs), the electronic version of a patient's medical history, including demographics, progress notes, problems, and medications, are maintained by a particular provider over time (Coventry & Branley, 2018).

Healthcare is vulnerable due to a historic lack of investment in cybersecurity, vulnerabilities in existing technology, and staff behaviour. Electronic health records, the healthcare infrastructure, and individual medical devices are all targets of cybercriminals. Breaches have resulted in millions of stolen health records and have on occasion brought the infrastructure to a standstill, which could have cost patient lives. Cybersecurity breaches might include health-related information and ransomware attacks on hospitals and medical institutions can lead to patient trust reduction.

In 2017, the WannaCry attack outbreak impacted the National Health Service (NHS) in the UK for several days, affecting hospitals and general practice (GP) surgeries across England and Scotland (NHS, 2018). The attack affected services such as ambulance despatch, out-of-hours appointment bookings, mental health services, and emergency prescriptions (Smart, 2018). However, since the beginning of the COVID-19 pandemic, we have witnessed a surge in reporting of cyberattacks on healthcare systems. It is certainly the case that, although some of these attacks have been extremely successful, defenders have thwarted some very significant attempts at compromising institutions within this sector.

Cybersecurity in healthcare has become a challenge due to the nature and sensitivity of medical data (Altynpara, 2022). There are a number of primary concerns for healthcare facilities (Deloitte, 2020) such as:

- **Phishing attacks:** Links or attachments in phishing emails, social media, or text messages infect computer systems with malware, which often spreads over the clinical network.

DOI: 10.4324/9781003364184-3

- **Man-in-the-middle (MITM) attacks:** Cybercriminals inject themselves into conversations or data transfers and steal confidential (and very valuable) user info, causing severe losses and penalties for a confidentiality breach.
- **Attacks to network vulnerabilities:** Address resolution protocol (ARP) cache poisoning, hypertext transfer protocol secure (HTTPS) spoofing, and other cybercrimes target the vital bastion of medical centres – wired and wireless networks, which provide access to patient information.
- **Ransomware attacks:** Criminals not only encrypt data and extort money for decryption but also block access to the entire clinical system, paralysing the work of equipment for surgical operations and life support.

In all health professions, including counselling and psychotherapy practice, ethical behaviour is essential. As a means of maintaining higher quality of therapeutic relationships, therapists need to make sure that the confidentiality of client information is always guaranteed in their face-to-face and online sessions, and this is why most therapists also express that they do not share client data with the helpdesk when technical issues transpire (Mol et al., 2019). However, not all therapists believe that online therapy, can be guaranteed as confidential or ethically effective compared to face-to-face sessions or traditional therapy.

Lucassen et al. (2015) stated that online session-interventions can be effective ethically when extra precaution and privacy is guaranteed. Regardless of this, Internet safety should always be considered by the user and this could mean there are still some risks of utilising the online platform from a client's or a therapist's perspective (Lucassen et al., 2018).

2 Confidentiality and patient data protection

Legislation and regulations are in place to facilitate change. Healthcare providers and their business partners have to balance protecting patient privacy, providing quality care, and complying with the Health Insurance Portability and Accountability Act (HIPAA, 1996) in the US and the General Data Protection Regulation (GDPR, 2018) in Europe. According to these, counselling and psychotherapy practitioners can disclose private information without the patient's or client's consent in order to protect the patient or the public from serious harm (e.g. suicide attempts); psychologists are required to report ongoing domestic violence, abuse, or neglect of children, the elderly, or people with disabilities, and may release information if they receive a court order.

Whether working with clients online or face-to-face, practitioners today increasingly rely on cyberspace as part of their practice (Lamont-Mills et al., 2018). The NHS in the UK (2013) published a guide to confidentiality in health and social care, focusing on treating confidential information with respect, in order to provide assurance to the client.

The British Association for Counselling and Psychotherapy (BACP) Ethical Framework states that[1] *'Being trustworthy – honouring the trust placed in the practitioner'*, and to '*show respect by protecting client confidentiality and privacy'* are key commitments to clients. The UK Council for Psychotherapy (UKCP)[2] recognises the need for confidentiality and identified that conducting therapy online brings particular issues of confidentiality, and particular attention is paid to security over the method of payment.

The British Psychological Society (BPS, 2022) provided guidance on the use of technology in psychological practice, including teletherapy and other forms of remote service delivery. Overall, the BPS guidance on the use of technology in psychological practice is similar to that of the American Psychological Association (APA), emphasising the importance of maintaining high standards of professionalism, competence, and ethics when using technology to deliver psychological services. By following these guidelines, psychologists can provide effective and ethical care to their clients while also protecting their confidentiality and privacy. Some of the key points from this guidance include:

- **Competence:** Psychologists are expected to have the necessary knowledge and skills to use technology in their practice effectively and ethically.
- **Informed consent:** Clients must be provided with clear and accurate information about the use of technology in their treatment, including the potential risks and benefits, and be given the opportunity to ask questions and provide informed consent.
- **Confidentiality and security:** Psychologists must take appropriate steps to ensure the confidentiality and security of client information, such as using secure communication platforms, implementing strong passwords and encryption, and regularly updating security software.
- **Boundaries:** Psychologists are expected to establish clear boundaries around the use of technology in their practice, such as specifying when and how they will communicate with clients and ensuring that they are available to respond to emergencies.
- **Record-keeping:** Psychologists must keep accurate and complete records of their use of technology in their practice, including the platforms and tools they use, the dates and times of communication, and any relevant discussions or agreements with clients.
- **Professionalism:** Psychologists are expected to maintain a professional demeanour when using technology in their practice, including dressing appropriately and ensuring that their workspace is free of distractions.
- **Crisis management:** Psychologists must have a plan in place for managing crisis situations that may arise during teletherapy or other forms of remote service delivery.
- **Considering the individual needs and circumstances of clients when using technology in psychological practice:** This includes ensuring that clients have access to the necessary technology and support to participate in teletherapy or other forms of remote service delivery, and taking steps to address any barriers or challenges that may arise.

Confidentiality is a respected part of psychology's code of ethics (APA, 2019, 2017). Psychologists understand that for people to feel comfortable talking about private and revealing information, they need a safe place to talk about anything they wish, without fear of that information leaving the room. The APA's (2017) guidance on the use of technology in psychological practice emphasises the importance of maintaining high standards of professionalism, competence, and ethics when using technology to deliver psychological services. By following these guidelines, psychologists can provide effective and ethical care to their clients while also protecting their patients' confidentiality and privacy.

The APA and the BPS both provide guidance on the use of technology in psychological practice, including teletherapy and other forms of remote service delivery. While there are some similarities in their recommendations, there are also some differences.

One of the main differences between the two organisations is that the APA's guidelines (2017) specifically address the use of telepsychology across state or national borders, while the BPS does not. In terms of informed consent, the APA recommends that psychologists obtain written consent specifically for telepsychology, while the BPS does not require written consent but recommends that psychologists discuss the risks and benefits of teletherapy with their clients and obtain their verbal consent. The APA (2019) also recommends that psychologists take steps to ensure the privacy and security of client information, including using encryption and secure Internet connections, while the BPS provides more general guidance on the importance of ensuring confidentiality and security but does not provide specific recommendations. Overall, whilst there are some differences between the APA's and BPS's guidance on teletherapy, both organisations emphasise the importance of ethical and professional practice, informed consent, confidentiality, and the use of technology to enhance the quality of care provided to clients.

With the introduction of the General Data Protection Regulation (GDPR), organisations and practitioners must ensure that they comply with the regulations to protect client data from unauthorised access, use, or disclosure. The main measures that need to be taken are:

- **Secure data storage:** One of the essential measures to ensure client confidentiality is to store client data securely. This involves using encryption, firewalls, access controls, and other security measures to prevent unauthorised access. The storage location must also be secure, with physical and logical access controls.
- **Limit access to data:** Employees should be given access only to the data that is necessary for them to perform their job duties. By limiting access to data, businesses can minimise the risk of data breaches and ensure client confidentiality.
- **Data Protection Impact Assessment (DPIA):** DPIA is a process that helps organisations identify and minimise privacy risks when processing personal data. It involves assessing the impact of data processing on the rights and freedoms of individuals and taking measures to mitigate the risks. DPIA must be carried out before processing personal data that presents a high risk to the rights and freedoms of individuals.

- **Privacy by design and default:** Privacy by design and default is an approach that seeks to embed privacy and data protection into the design and operation of systems, processes, and products. It involves considering privacy and data protection at every stage of the development lifecycle, from the initial design to the final disposal of data. Privacy by design and default can help organisations and practitioners to comply with GDPR and ensure client confidentiality.
- **Employee training:** Employees play a critical role in ensuring client confidentiality. Therefore, organisations must ensure that their employees receive regular training on data protection and cybersecurity best practices. Training should cover topics such as password management, phishing, social engineering, and physical security.
- **Data breach notification:** In the event of a data breach, businesses must notify the relevant authorities and affected individuals without undue delay. Under GDPR, businesses must notify the relevant supervisory authority within 72 hours of becoming aware of the breach. Failure to notify can result in fines and reputational damage.

2.1 Risks to patient/client confidentiality

Confidentiality is a core principle of psychotherapy, and it is essential for building trust and fostering an open and honest therapeutic relationship between the patient and the therapist. In traditional in-person therapy sessions, confidentiality is protected by the physical environment, with the therapist's office providing a private and secure setting for the patient to share their thoughts and feelings. However, in online psychotherapy sessions, confidentiality can be more challenging to maintain.

There are several potential avenues through which confidentiality breaches can occur, including: (a) *Unsecured communication channels*: If the communication channel used to conduct the session is not adequately secured, it can be intercepted by third parties, who can then access and potentially even manipulate the content of the communication; (b) *Hacking a therapist's computer*: If the therapist's computer is infected with malware, or if their online accounts are compromised; (c) *Data breaches at online platform providers*: If these platforms suffer a data breach, patient information can be accessed by unauthorised parties (Seh et al., 2020).

In addition, there are several risks to patient confidentiality and data security in the field of psychotherapy. Some of the key risks include:

- **Unauthorised access:** Psychotherapy records often contain sensitive and personal information about patients, including their mental health history, diagnoses, and treatment plans. Unauthorised access to this information could result in embarrassment, discrimination, or other negative consequences for the patient. This risk can occur due to a lack of access controls, such as weak passwords or sharing of login credentials.

- **Data breaches:** Data breaches can occur when psychotherapy records are accessed by unauthorised parties or when the records are stolen or lost. Data breaches can result in the loss or exposure of sensitive patient information, which can lead to identity theft or other negative consequences for the patient.
- **Malware attacks:** Psychotherapy practices often use EHR systems to store patient information. Malware attacks, such as ransomware or phishing attacks, can compromise these systems and result in the loss or exposure of patient information.
- **Human error:** Human error is another risk for patient confidentiality and data security in psychotherapy. For example, a therapist may accidentally send an email containing sensitive patient information to the wrong recipient, or leave a patient file open on their desk where it can be viewed by unauthorised individuals.
- **Lack of awareness:** Patients may not be aware of their rights regarding their mental health information and may not be aware of the risks associated with sharing this information. This can lead to patients unknowingly sharing sensitive information with individuals who may not have a legitimate need to know.

2.2 Examples of healthcare cyberattacks

Healthcare organisations have become a prime target for cyberattacks due to the sensitive and valuable nature of the information they store. There are a number of risks associated with confidentiality breaches in healthcare. In particular, when considering online psychotherapy, there have been a number of high-profile incidents in recent years that demonstrate the potential impact of these risks. Some examples of healthcare cyberattacks include the following.

Ransomware attacks

In a ransomware attack, a cybercriminal gains access to a healthcare organisation's systems and encrypts the data, effectively locking it down. The attacker then demands payment in exchange for the decryption key. In order to gain control of networks, malware is used and data is then exfiltrated before the original copy is encrypted. The ransom demand is then not only for the restoration of the data, which an organisation with good backups can ignore, but also for destroying the data copy rather than publishing it on the Internet, which can lead to serious reputational damage. The significant amounts of money, the sensitivity of data, and the importance of continued operation has made some healthcare sectors prime targets.

For example, in March 2020 a cyberattack took down the network of a Czech hospital that was also a COVID-19 testing laboratory (Guardian News and Media, 2020). In the same month a ransomware attack on a vaccine trial group in UK led to the publication of personal details of former patients, but it failed in its attempt to disable the network (Goodwin, 2020).

In 2018, a data breach at a third-party provider of online psychotherapy services in Finland resulted in the exposure of confidential patient information, including names, email addresses, and health information (Guardian News and Media,

2020). The breach affected over 150,000 patients, and the company faced significant reputational damage and regulatory scrutiny as a result. Shocked patients were then asked to pay individual Bitcoin ransoms to prevent the contents of their discussions with therapists being made public.

In September 2020, Universal Health Services (UHS), one of the largest hospital chains in the US, was hit by a ransomware attack. The attack caused widespread system outages and forced the company to shut down computer systems at its 400 facilities across the US (NBC Universal News Group, 2020). In May 2020, the non-profit fundraising software provider Blackbaud suffered a ransomware attack that affected several of its clients, including several healthcare organisations. The attackers stole sensitive information, including donor information, and threatened to publish it if the ransom was not paid (ITRC, 2020). In May 2021, Ireland's Health Service Executive (HSE) suffered a ransomware attack that caused widespread system outages and disrupted healthcare services across the country. The attackers demanded a ransom of $20 million in exchange for the decryption key (O'Connor, 2021).

Phishing attacks

In a phishing attack, cybercriminals use social engineering tactics, such as sending emails that appear to be from a trusted source, to trick healthcare employees into divulging sensitive information. Phishing attacks can lead to data breaches, which can be costly for healthcare organisations. A phishing attack can also lead to a ransomware attack. For example, in April 2021, Magellan Health, a US healthcare provider, suffered a data breach that affected the personal information of 365,000 patients. The breach was caused by a phishing attack on one of the company's employees (Davis, 2021).

DDoS attacks

In a distributed denial-of-service (DDoS) attack, cybercriminals flood a healthcare organisation's network with traffic, effectively causing it to shut down. This can prevent patients from accessing critical services, such as emergency care, and can disrupt the organisation's ability to provide care.

Insider threats

Not all cyberattacks are the work of outside actors. Insider threats can come from employees or contractors who intentionally or unintentionally access or share patient information. This can be especially damaging as the individuals responsible may have access to sensitive patient information.

Supply chain attacks

Healthcare organisations rely on a variety of vendors and third-party providers for their services. A supply chain attack occurs when a cybercriminal gains access to one of these providers and uses it as a way to access the healthcare organisation's systems.

Zoom-bombing

As the COVID-19 pandemic forced many mental health professionals to switch to virtual therapy sessions, Zoom has emerged as a popular platform for conducting online therapy sessions. However, the use of Zoom for therapy raises several concerns about data privacy and confidentiality. Zoom has faced criticism for its data privacy practices, including reports of data breaches, unauthorised data sharing, and lack of end-to-end encryption. These concerns are particularly relevant in the context of psychotherapy, where confidentiality and privacy are critical for building trust and facilitating therapeutic progress.

One major concern is the possibility of data breaches. Zoom has acknowledged several security vulnerabilities in the past, such as 'Zoom-bombing', where unauthorised individuals gain access to a meeting and disrupt the session. While Zoom has implemented measures to address these vulnerabilities, such incidents highlight the potential for breaches of client confidentiality and the importance of ensuring that virtual therapy sessions are conducted in a secure and private environment (O'Flaherty, 2020).

Another concern is the lack of end-to-end encryption, a security measure which ensures that only the sender and recipient can access the contents of a message, and not any intermediaries, including the service provider. In the context of online psychotherapy, end-to-end encryption is crucial for protecting client confidentiality and preventing unauthorised access to session data. However, Zoom's initial implementation of encryption did not provide end-to-end encryption, which raised concerns about the security of confidential client information.

Moreover, Zoom has been accused of sharing data with third-party services, including Facebook and LinkedIn, without user consent (Lee & Grauer, 2020). This data sharing includes personal data and may potentially compromise client confidentiality. Even if Zoom claims that this sharing has been halted, the possibility of *un*authorised data sharing still raises concerns about the privacy of virtual therapy sessions.

Finally, there is the risk of technical issues, such as poor video and audio quality, or dropped connections. Technical issues can disrupt the flow of therapy sessions and undermine the therapeutic relationship. They can also lead to client frustration and dissatisfaction with the therapeutic process.

Mental health professionals and clinicians need to be aware of these risks and take steps to ensure that virtual therapy sessions are conducted in a secure and private environment. This may include using a secure video conferencing platform that offers end-to-end encryption, obtaining client consent for the use of the platform, and implementing measures to address potential technical issues. By prioritising data privacy and confidentiality, mental health professionals can ensure that virtual therapy sessions are effective and ethical.

Zoom has responded to these concerns and has taken steps to improve its data privacy and security practices (The Verge, 2020). However, these reports highlight the importance of being aware of potential data privacy risks and taking steps to protect confidential information during online therapy sessions.

These are just a few examples of cyberattacks on healthcare organisations. The healthcare industry remains a prime target for cybercriminals, and it is essential for organisations to take steps to protect their systems and patient data.

3 Mitigating risks

It is important to note that many of these risks can be mitigated with proper precautions and safeguards. Healthcare organisations can ensure patient confidentiality and data security by implementing access controls, encryption, secure communication channels, regular security audits, employee training, and compliance with regulations. By taking these steps they can protect sensitive patient data from unauthorised access and potential breaches, which helps to maintain patient trust and protect their privacy.

There are several measures that healthcare organisations and practitioners can take to ensure patient confidentiality and data security, including:

- **Access controls:** Healthcare organisations can implement access controls that require users to log in with a unique username and password to access sensitive patient data. Additionally, access controls can be used to limit access to certain data based on an individual's job role or level of clearance.
- **Encryption:** Encryption is the process of encoding sensitive data to protect it from unauthorised access. Healthcare organisations can use encryption to protect sensitive patient data both in transit and at rest. This can include encrypting data stored on servers, laptops, and other mobile devices, as well as encrypting data transmitted over networks.
- **Secure communication channels:** Healthcare organisations can use secure communication channels, such as secure email, virtual private networks (VPNs), and secure messaging apps, to securely share sensitive patient data. This can help prevent unauthorised access and potential breaches.
- **Regular security audits:** Healthcare organisations should conduct regular security audits to identify potential vulnerabilities and risks to patient confidentiality and data security. These can include conducting penetration testing, vulnerability scans, and security risk assessments.
- **Employee training:** Healthcare organisations should provide ongoing employee training to ensure that all employees are aware of the importance of patient confidentiality and data security. This can include training on best practices for securing patient data, how to identify potential security threats, and how to report suspected security incidents.
- **Compliance with regulations:** Healthcare organisations must comply with various regulations, such as the Health Insurance Portability and Accountability Act (HIPAA), that require them to protect patient confidentiality and data security. Compliance with these regulations is essential to ensure that patient data is protected from unauthorised access and potential breaches.

4 Ten ways to protect patient confidentiality and data security

By implementing security measures, psychotherapy practices can help protect patient confidentiality and data security and maintain patient trust. It is essential for practices to stay up-to-date on emerging threats and technologies and to continually reassess their security measures to ensure they remain effective in protecting patient information. Changes are required to human behaviour, technology, and processes as part of a holistic solution. Moving forward, cybersecurity must be an integral part of the patient care pathway.

More specifically, for online psychotherapy, therapists can use secure online platforms that are designed specifically for and take steps to ensure the privacy and security of patient information. To mitigate the risks associated with confidentiality breaches in online psychotherapy, it is important to take a number of precautions. These include:

1 **Using secure communication channels:** Online psychotherapy sessions should be conducted using secure communication channels that are encrypted and protected from interception by unauthorised parties. The use of secure channels helps to ensure that the content of the communication is protected, even if the channel is intercepted. Public Wi-Fi networks can allow hackers access to any computer that connects with them.

2 **Implementing access controls:** For example, strong passwords and two-factor authentication.

3 **Encrypting patient data both at rest and in transit:** To protect data in transit and at rest, network security controls like firewalls and network access control can be implemented. These will protect the networks used against cyberattacks.

4 **Regularly backing up patient data:** To prevent data loss in the event of a breach or other disaster.

5 **Protecting the therapist's computer:** Therapists should take steps to protect their computer and online accounts from hacking and other forms of compromise. This can include using up-to-date antivirus software, regularly changing passwords, and being mindful of phishing attacks and other forms of social engineering.

6 **Educating patients and employees about privacy and security:** Patients should be educated about the risks associated with online psychotherapy and the measures they can take to protect their own privacy and security. This can include using a secure Internet connection, avoiding public Wi-Fi networks, and being mindful of the information they share during online sessions. Similarly, there should be regular training for staff on best practices for protecting patient confidentiality and data security.

7 **Choosing secure online platform providers:** When selecting a third-party provider to conduct online psychotherapy sessions, it is important to choose a provider that has a strong track record of protecting patient data and maintaining high levels of security. Providers should be transparent about their

security practices and provide clear information about the measures they take to protect patient confidentiality.

8 **Ensuring that third-party vendors who have access to patient information have appropriate security measures in place.**

9 **Regularly conducting security risk assessments:** To identify potential vulnerabilities and risks.

10 **Establishing clear policies and procedures for handling patient information:** To include data retention and destruction.

Notes

1 BACP. Confidentiality resources – Ethical Framework for the Counselling Professions. https://www.bacp.co.uk/events-and-resources/ethics-and-standards/ethical-framework-for-the-counselling-professions/confidentiality/

2 UK Council for Psychotherapy (UKCP). Practice policy 4: Confidentiality. https://www.psychotherapy.org.uk/media/zaqe1esm/csrp-practice-policy-4_confidentiality.pdf

References

Altynpara, E. (2022, 14 April). Council post: Cybersecurity and data protection in healthcare. Forbes. Retrieved 26 February 2023, from https://www.forbes.com/sites/forbestechcouncil/2022/02/15/cybersecurity-and-data-protection-in-healthcare/?sh=17f8acd65048.

APA. (2017). Ethical principles of psychologists and code of conduct. American Psychological Association. Retrieved 26 February 2023, from https://www.apa.org/ethics/code.

APA. (2019). Protecting your privacy: Understanding confidentiality. American Psychological Association. Retrieved 26 February 2023, from https://www.apa.org/topics/psychotherapy/confidentiality.

BACP. Confidentiality resources – Ethical framework for the counselling professions. Retrieved 26 February 2023, from https://www.bacp.co.uk/events-and-resources/ethics-and-standards/ethical-framework-for-the-counselling-professions/confidentiality/.

BPS. (2022). Effective therapy via video: Top tips. Retrieved 26 February 2023, from https://cms.bps.org.uk/sites/default/files/2022-06/Effective%20therapy%20via%20video%20-%20top%20tips.pdf.

Coventry, L., & Branley, D. (2018). Cybersecurity in healthcare: A narrative review of trends, threats and ways forward. *Maturitas, 113*, 48–52.

Davis, J. (2021, 19 October). Magellan Health Data Breach Victim Tally reaches 365K patients. HealthITSecurity. Retrieved 26 February 2023, from https://healthitsecurity.com/news/magellan-health-data-breach-victim-tally-reaches-365k-patients.

Deloitte (2020, 14 December). Data privacy and cybersecurity in the future of health. Retrieved 26 February 2023, from https://www2.deloitte.com/us/en/pages/advisory/articles/data-privacy-and-cybersecurity-in-the-future-of-health.html.

GDPR (2018). Retrieved 26 February 2023, from https://gdpr-info.eu.

Goodwin, B. (2020, 22 March). Cyber gangsters hit UK medical firm poised for work on coronavirus with Maze Ransomware Attack. *ComputerWeekly.com*. Retrieved 26 February 2023, from https://www.computerweekly.com/news/252480425/Cyber-gangsters-hit-UK-medical-research-lorganisation-poised-for-work-on-Coronavirus.

Guardian News and Media. (2020, 3 May). Hostile states trying to steal coronavirus research, says UK agency. *The Guardian*. Retrieved 26 February 2023, from https://www.theguardian.com/world/2020/may/03/hostile-states-trying-to-steal-coronavirus-research-says-uk-agency.

Guardian News and Media. (2020, 26 October). 'Shocking' hack of psychotherapy records in Finland affects thousands. *The Guardian*. Retrieved 26 February 2023, from https://www.theguardian.com/world/2020/oct/26/tens-of-thousands-psychotherapy-records-hacked-in-finland.

HIPAA. (1996). The standard for sensitive patient data protection. Retrieved 26 February 2023, from https://www.hhs.gov/hipaa/index.html.

ITRC. (2020, 3 May). Blackbaud data breach leaves lasting impact on US and international nonprofits. Retrieved 26 February 2023, from https://www.idtheftcenter.org/post/blackbaud-data-breach-leaves-lasting-impact-on-u-s-and-international-nonprofits/.

Kioskli, K., Fotis, T., & Mouratidis, H. (2021, August). *The landscape of cybersecurity vulnerabilities and challenges in healthcare: Security standards and paradigm shift recommendations.* In Proceedings of the 16th International Conference on Availability, Reliability and Security (pp. 1–9).

Lamont-Mills, A., Christensen, S., & Moses, L. (2018). Confidentiality and informed consent in counselling and psychotherapy: A systematic review. Melbourne: PACFA. Retrieved 26 February 2023, from https://www.pacfa.org.au/common/Uploaded%20files/PCFA/Documents/Research/Confidentiality-and-informed-consent-in-counselling-and-psychotherapy-a-systematic-review.pdf.

Lee, M., & Grauer, Y. (2020, 31 March). Zoom meetings aren't end-to-end encrypted, despite misleading marketing. The Intercept. Retrieved 26 February 2023, from https://theintercept.com/2020/03/31/zoom-meeting-encryption/.

Lucassen, M.F., Merry, S.N., Hatcher, S., & Frampton, C.M. (2015). Rainbow SPARX: A novel approach to addressing depression in sexual minority youth. *Cognitive and Behavioural Practice, 22(2)*, 203–216.

Lucassen, M., Samra, R., Iacovides, I., Fleming, T., Shepherd, M., Stasiak, K., & Wallace, L. (2018). How LGBT+ young people use the internet in relation to their mental health and envisage the use of e-therapy: Exploratory study. *JMIR Serious Games, 6(4)*, e11249.

Mol, M., van Genugten, C., Dozeman, E., van Schaik, D.J., Draisma, S., Riper, H., & Smit, J. H. (2019). Why uptake of blended internet-based interventions for depression is challenging: A qualitative study on therapists' perspectives. *Journal of Clinical Medicine, 9(1)*, 91.

NBC Universal News Group. (2020, 28 September). Major hospital system hit with cyberattack, potentially largest in U.S. history. NBCNews.com. Retrieved 26 February 2023, from https://www.nbcnews.com/tech/security/cyberattack-hits-major-u-s-hospital-system-n1241254.

NHS. (2013). A guide to confidentiality in health and social care: Treating confidential information with respect. Retrieved 26 February 2023, from https://digital.nhs.uk/data-and-information/looking-after-information/data-security-and-information-governance/codes-of-practice-for-handling-information-in-health-and-care/a-guide-to-confidentiality-in-health-and-social-care/a-guide-to-confidentiality.

NHS England. (2018). *Lessons learned: Review of the WannaCry ransomware cyber attack.* Retrieved 26 February 2023, from https://www.england.nhs.uk/wp-content/uploads/2018/02/lessons-learned-review-wannacry-ransomware-cyber-attack-cio-review.pdf.

O'Connor, N. (2021, 21 May). HSE ransomware attack began on a single computer when an employee clicked on a link. *The Journal.ie*. Retrieved 26 February 2023, from https://www.thejournal.ie/hse-cyber-attack-ransomware-started-5443370-May2021/.

O'Flaherty, K. (2020, 28 June). Beware zoom users: Here's how people can 'zoom-bomb' your chat. Forbes. Retrieved 26 February 2023, from https://www.forbes.com/sites/kateoflaher tyuk/2020/03/27/beware-zoom-users-heres-how-people-can-zoom-bomb-your-chat/?sh =53bbdad7618e.

Seh, A.H., Zarour, M., Alenezi, M., Sarkar, A.K., Agrawal, A., Kumar, R., & Ahmad Khan, R. (2020). Healthcare data breaches: Insights and implications. *Healthcare*, *8*(2), 133. MDPI AG. Retrieved from http://dx.doi.org/10.3390/healthcare8020133.

Smart, W. (2018). Lessons learned review of the Wannacry ransomware cyber attack. Department of Health and Social Care. Retrieved 26 February 2023, from https:// www.england.nhs.uk/wp-content/uploads/2018/02/lessons-learned-review-wanna cry-ransomware-cyber-attack-cio-review.pdf.

The Verge (2020). Zoom promises to address privacy and security issues as use soars. Retrieved 26 February 2023, from https://www.theverge.com/2020/4/1/21202809/ zoom-privacy-security-issues-apology-fixes-plan.

3   Data protection and the GDPR

Why there is more than one legislation you must know

Philip Brining

Introduction

Data protection: What does it mean? To some it means doing things to protect data. Cybersecurity, for instance, and, to others, it means the legal framework of privacy laws, perhaps the Data Protection Act. This chapter focuses on the latter meaning and outlines some of the aspects of the law that affect the collection and handling of information about patients by clinicians.

Background to the law

It is likely that the discussion and debate about the protection of privacy goes back a very long way into the depths of humanity's history. Data protection is perhaps a more modern phenomenon, the concept of 'data' being a prerequisite to thoughts of protecting it. However, traces of a legislative framework for the protection of data go back further than many people expect. Some of the key moments are plotted below and are useful to consider, as this provides an informed context for where we are today.

In 1710, the Post Office (Revenues) Act (25 November 1710) established a postal service in the British colonies and set out offences, such as opening, delaying, or detaining letters or packets sent in the mail. In essence, this was about protecting privacy: providing a legal framework for protecting information stored and transmitted via a communications system on the medium of paper. Over a century later, eminent US lawyers Warren and Brandeis published a paper (Warren & Brandeis, 1890) in which they wrote that the law should protect privacy as well as property and concluded that individuals surely must have the right 'to be let alone'. Consider the timing. Warren and Brandeis's work came hot on the heels of developments in photography where a new type of information was being collected, stored, and distributed. Warren and Brandeis's work remains an insightful read 100-plus years on.

Legislation to regulate the access to and use of information was introduced in the UK shortly afterwards, when, having discovered that secret plans of British naval battleships had been sold to overseas powers, the government of the day was astonished that such behaviour was not illegal. It is unlikely there is any

DOI: 10.4324/9781003364184-4

connection between Warren and Brandeis's work and the Official Secrets Act (1898) but, just as Warren and Brandeis's thoughts were likely stimulated by the development and use of technology, the Official Secrets Act (1898) was enacted as a reaction to events. We are reminded that the law is a social construct influenced by factors such as politics, economics, and technology.

Those who work with the General Data Protection Regulation (GDPR) (see EU Regulation 2016/679 of the European Parliament and of the Council of 27 April 2016 on the protection of natural persons with regard to the processing of personal data and on the free movement of such data), the legislative regime introduced across the European Union (EU) in 2016, will no doubt be familiar with references to the 'fundamental rights and freedoms' of data subjects, natural persons, or individuals. The phrase 'rights and freedoms' in fact occurs 70 times in the GDPR and is one of its cornerstones. But what does it mean?

The notion of 'fundamental rights and freedoms' stems from the 1950 European Convention of Human Rights (ECHR). Article 8 of the ECHR declared that 'everyone has the right to respect for his private and family life, his home and his correspondence'; i.e. the right to privacy and, by extension, the protection of data that could impact privacy. Each time the GDPR (EU or UK versions) refers to 'fundamental rights and freedoms', it is in fact referencing at least Article 8 of the ECHR. It probably goes without saying that the development of the concept of human rights and enshrining them in international agreements followed the horrors of the Second World War.

In Britain, during the 1960s, several private members' bills regarding privacy and the protection of data were put before the UK parliament. The transcripts of parliamentary debates suggest that initially the drivers for these bills were efforts to curb what was perceived as an intrusive press. For example, Lord Mancroft's address during the second reading of his Right of Privacy Bill in 1961 is critical of the press's harrying of Manchester United players after the Munich air crash, and Her Royal Highness Princess Margaret among others. But the focus of these Bills and the associated public narrative markedly changed in the late 1960s. Kenneth Baker's Data Surveillance Bill of 1969, and Lord Windlesham's Computers and Personal Records Bill of 1969 heralded the advancement of computer technologies. The reports of the Younger and Lindop Committees (1972 and 1978 respectively) (Report of Committee on Privacy, 1972; and Report of the Committee on Data Protection, 1978, respectively) show a sophistication of thinking well beyond the Bills of the early 1960s and reflect a gathering of momentum behind the notion of the right to privacy and the protection of data relating to people. Key features of these reports were, in the case of Younger, setting out ten data protection principles; and, in the Lindop Report, the recommendation to establish an information commissioner.

In 1981 both the Organisation for Economic Cooperation and Development (OECD) and the Council of Europe published guidelines on data protection and privacy. The OECD guidelines (OECD, 23 September 1980) focused on transborder flows of personal data, while the Council of Europe's Convention 108 (1980) were more rights oriented. Under Convention 108, the signatories were required to take the necessary steps in their domestic legislation to apply the principles it laid down, in order to ensure respect in their territory for the fundamental human rights of all individuals with regard to processing of personal data. This acted as a prompt for European countries to put in place data protection and privacy legislation.

In the UK, the social and economic backdrop of the early Thatcher years (1979–1983) had arguably put the work of Younger, Lindop, and others onto the back burner. And once European countries began to sign up to Convention 108, concern grew that if the UK did not have any data protection legislation, countries that had ratified the Convention would prohibit the transfer of personal data to countries that had not. This meant that, without data protection legislation in the UK, personal data could be withheld from the City of London's vital financial centres with the lack of UK data protection legislation cited as the reason. In the early 1980s, with the structural changes to the UK economy implemented by the Thatcher government, this would have had devastating consequences. Thus, the Data Protection Act (1984) was passed.

During the German reunification process between 1989 and 1991, public awareness about the data collected and used by the Stasi in East Germany increased the demand for privacy in Germany. West Germany had enjoyed privacy laws since 1977 (BDSG 27 January 1977) and it became increasingly obvious to the European Commission that divergent data protection legislation among EU member states would impede the free flow of data within the EU. Accordingly, the Data Protection Directive was enacted in 1995 (Directive 95/46/EC 1995) which, as a Directive, required each member state to enact domestic legislation to bring the Directive into effect. In the UK, that manifested itself as the Data Protection Act 1998.

The data protection directive was designed to protect personal data stored on computers or in an organised paper filing system. Its aim was to enable the free flow of data between member states while providing protection to the rights and freedoms of data subjects.

The meteoric growth of electronic communications in the late twentieth century and beginning of the twenty-first century led to legislation to regulate telecommunications and Internet services. The European e-Privacy Directive (12 July 2002), complements the general data protection regime and sets out more specific privacy rights with regard to electronic communications, including security of telecommunications transmissions, as well as rules about direct marketing by phone, fax, and electronic messaging. A 2011 revision regulated the use of cookies (Directive 2009/136/EC).

In October 2013, Phillip Albrecht, a German politician, MEP, and member of the European Parliament's Committee on Civil Liberties (LIBE), put forward a proposal for a general EU-wide data protection regulation that was adopted by LIBE (https://www.europarl.europa.eu/doceo/document/A-7-2013-0402_EN.html). Albrecht led the negotiations between the European Parliament and the Council of Ministers on the adoption of the regulation and, after lengthy discussion, a deal was reached in December 2015 and the GDPR was adopted by Council and Parliament in April 2016.

As a regulation, (as opposed to a directive), the GDPR was directly applicable in all 28 member states. It did not require any domestic implementing legislation and took immediate, direct effect. It replaced the pre-existing directive-based data protection law in all 28 member states.

At the same time that the GDPR was enacted, the EU enacted the EU Law Enforcement Directive (Directive (EU) 2016/680) (LED). This directive complemented the GDPR, which specifically excludes data processing by law enforcement and intelligence services (GDPR, Articles 2(2)(b) and 2(2)(c), page 32). As a directive, the LED required implementing through domestic legislation and, in the UK, the Data Protection Act 2018 (DPA18) did just that. The DPA18 also expanded on and clarified certain aspects of the GDPR as it applied to the UK and contains some important points for the clinical practitioner.

With Brexit came more change but, essentially, the UK GDPR (United Kingdom General Data Protection Regulation) [2016] No. 679) is a copy of the EU GDPR (EU Regulation 2016/679), albeit with EU references replaced or removed. At the time of writing there is talk of further reform to the UK data protection regime. Time will tell how the next moves pan out.

In this chapter the term 'GDPR', references the UK GDPR but the comments apply equally to the EU GDPR.

For the practitioner

For today's practitioner, the UK GDPR and Data Protection Act (2018) provide the main legislative framework. The Privacy and Electronic Communications Regulations (2003) provide additional regulation about the sending of unsolicited direct marketing by email, phone, and other electronic methods, and for the reading and writing data from/to users' devices, such as phones and computers (for example, using, placing and reading cookies).

The UK GDPR is the main piece of legislation for most of us, setting out a pretty straightforward set of rules of engagement. It easy to read and to follow and it is possible for a non-legal person to pick up a copy, read it, and gain an understanding of its requirements. It is far from prescriptive and leaves a lot open to interpretation. It has to. It is designed to provide a framework for all processing of all personal data across all sectors of the entire EU! It has to have 'wriggle room' in order to work. But often that is where people find it hard to work with, as they want certainty. They want to be told what they can and cannot do. They don't like having to make decisions when there is no clarity as to whether they have made the right decision.

Principles of data protection

The GDPR sets out seven principles (GDPR, Article 5, p. 35), which underpin everything. It is remarkable how similar they are to the principles proposed by the Younger Report's ten principles back in the 1970s. The seven principles are:

1   Fairness, lawfulness, and transparency.
2   Processing for defined purposes.
3   Using the minimal amount of data possible to achieve the processing objectives.
4   Ensuring that data are accurate and up-to-date.
5   Retaining data in a format where people are directly identifiable from it for as short a period of time as possible.
6   Ensuring that data are processed securely.
7   Being able to demonstrate that the principles above have been effectively implemented.

These principles can be applied to every data protection/privacy situation, and thinking about how any processing activity complies with them is a good starting point for checking if that processing activity is likely to be compliant. For example, when considering whether to disclose information about someone to another person, it is useful to work through the principles above. Would it be fair to make the disclosure? What is the lawful basis for the disclosure? How much information needs to be disclosed in order to achieve the aim of the disclosure? Is the information being disclosed likely to have a negative impact on the person it is about if it is wrong? How should the disclosure be made for it to be made securely? And what should be recorded to be able to evidence that the principles were considered?

Can I do …?

One of the most common questions asked of me as a data protection practitioner is 'am I allowed to do …?'. Contrary to popular opinion, there are very few things that the GDPR actually says you cannot do. Remember, its stated aim is the free movement of data. Most of the time the GDPR suggests that you can do something provided you put appropriate controls in place. Those controls include taking a risk-based approach, maintaining security of data, establishing a framework of policies and procedures to define acceptable approaches to data processing, and training people in the application of that framework. These are some of the core obligations incumbent on data controllers.

The concept of fair processing set out in the first principle refers to the need to tell people what you are intending to do with information relating to them (i.e. 'their personal data'). This is more about why data are being processed than how. Fairness is operationalised through the provision of privacy information, often referred to as privacy notices, or sometimes privacy policies, and the GDPR specifies what information must be provided to individuals (GDPR, Articles 13 and 14, pp. 40–42). This means that it is easy to test if privacy information is compliant.

The notion of transparency is an elaboration on the principle of fairness. A privacy notice must be truthful, complete, and not written in a way that is difficult to understand. Transparency is about being open and honest with those whose personal data you are processing or intending to process.

The lawfulness element of the first principle is linked to the second principle: that of processing only for specified, explicit, and legitimate purposes. The lawful basis for processing is a function of why you are processing it in the first place.

The GPDR provides six bases (GDPR, Article 6, pp. 36–37) that make the subsequent processing of personal data lawful. In summary these are:

1   **Consent:** Where the individual has given their consent to the processing of their personal data for one or more specific purposes.
2   **Contract:** Where the processing is necessary for the performance of a contract to which the data subject is party or in order to take steps at the request of the data subject prior to entering into a contract.
3   **Legal obligation:** Where the processing is necessary for the controller to comply with a legal obligation to which it is subject.
4   **Vital interests:** Where processing is necessary to protect someone's life that is in immediate danger.
5   **Public tasks:** Where the processing is necessary for the performance of a task carried out in the public interest or in the exercise of official authority vested in the controller.
6   **Legitimate interests:** Where the processing is necessary for the purposes of the legitimate interests pursued by the controller or by a third party, except where such interests are overridden by the interests or fundamental rights and freedoms of the data subject that require protection of personal data.

As a clinician you may be processing on the basis of consent but that is not the only lawful basis for processing. You may have a contract with your patient and processing personal data might be necessary for you to fulfil that contract. Or you may be processing personal data on the basis of authority vested in you through health-related legislation. The point really is that you can process personal data provided you do it in accordance with the data protection principles, i.e. providing you do it for specified purposes, fairly, transparently, and on the basis of one of the grounds or bases set out in the law, using the minimum amount of data that you keep up-to-date, only as long as is necessary and in an appropriately secure manner.

In terms of processing activities, it's generally the data protection principles that govern whether you can do something or not. There are other factors that need to be considered, which this chapter highlights, but in general the answer to the question, 'Can I do …?' is often, 'Yes, provided you do xyz'.

What is personal data?

Take a moment to consider what it is that the law is trying to regulate: the processing of personal data. The definition of processing encompasses pretty much anything you can do with data: collecting, storing, disclosing, sharing, destroying, transporting, viewing (GDPR, Article 4(2), p. 33) – any action you can envisage doing with or to data is classified as 'processing'.

The definition of 'personal data' is a little more complex but essentially it is information about a person (GDPR, Article 4(1), p. 33). An entire book could be written about the definition of personal data as it is subject to much legal debate, however suffice to say that some information is easier than others for us to identify as personal data. A medical record, for example, contains a host of information about a specific individual, the patient. It might contain information to identify them – such as their name, date of birth, or National Health Service number. It might contain information for the purposes of identity verification – such as a pass code, pass phrase, or PIN. It will contain information to enable you to contact and communicate with them – such as a postal address, email address, and phone number. It will contain information about their health, and information used to diagnose a medical condition perhaps, or information about a treatment plan, appointments, referrals, opinions of other medical professionals, results of scans, images, and so on. It might also contain information about their satisfaction with the services they have used and information about other people – such as those giving or managing treatment, emergency contact details for friends and relatives, and the like.

Broadly speaking *all* the information about the people who can be identified from the medical record is personal data about them. So, at the very least, a patient medical record is likely to contain a variety of different types of personal data about several people, which may be used for a variety of purposes.

You may often hear people use the term 'personally identifiable information' or 'PII'. Some may see this as a trendy 'moniker' for 'personal data'. A phrase that trips off the tongue more easily or perhaps does a better job of describing what it actually is. But we need to be aware that PII is an American term defined in US legislation (see US GSA Directive (2019) CIO P 2180.2 s. PII, https://www.gsa. gov/directive/gsa-rules-of-behavior-for-handling-personally-identifiable-information-(pii)) and standards (https://csrc.nist.gov/glossary/term/PII).   PII is not the same as personal data, and if you use the term PII, or personally identifiable information, you need to be aware that it might mean different things to different audiences.

Special categories of personal data

Any personal data that reveals the racial or ethnic origin, political opinions, religious or philosophical beliefs, or trade union membership of an individual are classified as 'special categories of personal data' as are genetic data and biometric data used for the purpose of uniquely identifying someone. In addition, data concerning health and data concerning someone's sex life or sexual orientation are also categorised as special categories of personal data (GDPR, Article 9, p. 38).

People working in the medical and health sector will undoubtedly process special categories of personal data: it is inevitable. 'Data concerning health' includes information about or related to a person's physical or mental health. It also includes information about the provision of healthcare services that reveal information about their health status. So, an invoice addressed to a patient for mental health counselling services might well be considered to contain special categories of personal data, as it at least infers if not reveals that the addressee is subject to a healthcare programme related to their mental health. If the invoice details aspects of the treatment plan, it may well also reveal the status of an individual's mental health.

The GDPR prohibits the processing of special categories of personal data without there being more specific lawful grounds. These are set out in Article 9(2) of the GDPR (Article 9(2), pp. 38–39) and include explicit consent and processing necessary for purposes of preventive or occupational medicine that may well be appropriate in a clinical setting.

'Explicit consent' differs from 'consent' only in so far as the data controller must ensure that it has provided specific and explicit information about the processing of the special category data in order to ensure that the consent is adequately informed. People need to be clear about what they are consenting to and give a positive, active indication of their consent. In practice this means that they generally will need somehow to show their agreement to a written statement about the proposed processing of their personal data. 'I consent to ..., etc., etc.' Note that it is the processing of their personal data that they are consenting to in the context of data protection law, as distinct from consenting to anything else (for example, a medical intervention. Consent for processing cannot be explicit if it is bundled up with consent for other things.

For the avoidance of doubt, a data controller is the person or organisation who either alone or jointly determines the means (i.e. the methods) and the purposes of processing (GDPR, Article 4(7), p. 33). In health settings, the data controller could be a health organisation or an individual medical practitioner – or both! A self-employed psychological wellbeing practitioner will be a data controller in the eyes of the law and therefore fully responsible for complying with the GDPR.

Lawful processing of special categories of personal data

The GDPR allows special categories of personal data to be processed where it is necessary for the purposes of preventive or occupational medicine (GDPR, Article 9 (2)(h), p. 38), providing the processing is carried out by a health professional or other person who is subject to the obligation of professional secrecy established in law or a competent body such as a National Health Service Trust. The nature of processing expressly permitted includes processing necessary for the assessment of an individual's capacity to work and processing necessary to perform a medical diagnosis. Processing necessary for the provision of health or social care or treatment is also expressly called out in the GDPR as being permitted. Finally, processing necessary for the management of health or social care systems and services is also provided for.

This list of permitted processing is broad but does not fully encompass the range of processing that a medical practitioner or clinician might encounter; and the GDPR also provides for a range of other lawful bases for processing special categories of personal data where processing is necessary for reasons of substantial public interest, provided such substantial public interest is set out in legislation (GDPR, Article 9(g), p. 38).

Helpfully, Schedule 1 of the Data Protection Act (2018) (DPA 2018, Sch. 1, pp. 131–147) provides a legal framework for processing carried out for reasons of substantial public interest in the UK. For example, the DPA18 sets out that processing certain special categories of personal data without consent (e.g. racial or ethnic background or sexual orientation) is lawful where processing is necessary for ensuring the equality of opportunity (DPA 2018, Sch.1 s. 8, p. 133). There are some specific conditions and restrictions around this but the point being made is that processing special categories of personal data without consent is, in certain cases, entirely lawful.

In the care setting, two particular, substantial public interest conditions for lawful processing are much relied upon. To illustrate the point, consider that you want to disclose personal data and special categories of personal data with another person. You need to think about whether the disclosure would be fair. Is it something that the data subject would reasonably expect you to do? Have you told them the types of disclosures you might make? The types of people to whom you might disclose information about them? The reason(s) or purposes of the disclosure? This is where privacy information can make the processing, in this case a disclosure to a third party, fair.

When it comes to ensuring that the processing (i.e. the disclosure) is lawful, you need to consider the lawful bases available to you. You could make the disclosure on the basis of the consent of the data subject, or explicit consent for the special categories of data you wish to disclose. But what if it is not possible or appropriate to obtain consent? What if such a disclosure might actually aggravate a delicate situation or what it if might result in significant detriment or harm to the data subject? What if they refuse? This is where understanding that there are lawful grounds for processing other than consent is vital.

As a clinician, the law would 'allow' (to use the vernacular) you to disclose medical information about a patient to another person without the patient's consent if you had reasonable cause to suspect that the individual had, for example, needs for care and support, was experiencing or was at risk of neglect or physical, mental, or emotional harm, and if, as a result of those needs, was unable to protect themselves against the neglect or the harm or the risk of it. The provisions that permit such processing of special categories of personal data (DPA 2018, Sch. 1 s. 18, p. 138) without consent understandably are set at a high bar, but in a clinical or social care setting, the circumstances that make such processing lawful are, sadly, all too readily prevalent.

The medical practitioner or clinician should probably seek advice from their data protection officer if they are in any doubt as to the lawfulness of any processing activities. However, a good rule of thumb is that if it seems sensible and reasonable to process data in a particular way for a particular purpose, then it is likely that the law makes provision for it. The role of the privacy practitioner is to help identify the correct lawful basis and to highlight any conditions surrounding it.

Other key elements of the GDPR

The GDPR sets out a series of rights bestowed upon data subjects and other individuals. There are four types of rights, some of which directly relate to the

Articles of the ECHR and others that give effect to the right to privacy. The four types of rights are:

1 The right to information about data processing activities (GDPR, Articles 13 and 14, pp. 40–42).
2 Rights relating to the personal data itself (e.g. the right of access, rectification, erasure, and portability) (GDPR, Articles 15 to 17, 19, and 20, pp. 43–45).
3 Rights relating to processing activities, e.g. the right to object to and to restrict processing activities (GDPR, Article 21 and 18, pp. 44–46), the right to withdraw consent for processing (GDPR, Article 7(3), p. 37), the right to the cessation of direct marketing (GDPR, Articles 21(2) and 21(3), p. 45), and the right to have a human review any automated decision making that has a significant effect on a data subject (GDPR, Article 22, p. 46).
4 Rights to remedies including compensation (GDPR, Article 82(1), p. 81), to complain to the Information Commissioners Office (ICO) (GDPR, Article 77, p. 80), and the right to take certain matters to the courts for a judicial remedy (GDPR, Articles 78–79, p. 80).

The Data Protection Act 2018 provides a host of exemptions that data controllers may rely on and which override people's rights (DPA 2018, Sch. 2, pp 147–164). For example, there are circumstances where personal data may be processed without informing the data subject, which would otherwise be unfair processing but for the DPA18 exemption.

The last key components of the GDPR directly affecting data controllers and processing are the articles which set out several obligations (GDPR, Articles 24–39, pp. 47–37 and Articles 44–49, pp. 60–65). In essence these provide a governance framework designed to ensure the free movement of data can happen in a controlled, structured, safe, and unintrusive manner. These obligations include:

- The requirement to notify the ICO and potentially data subjects of personal data breaches (GPDR 2018, Article 33, pp. 52–52).
- The requirement to undertake risk assessments for processing that might present a high risk to people's rights and freedoms, known as data protection impact assessments (DPIAs) or privacy impact assessments (PIAs) (GPDR 2018, Article 35, p. 53–54).
- The requirement not to transfer or allow the transfer of personal data outside the UK without suitable safeguards being in place (GPDR 2018, Articles 44–49, pp. 60–65).
- The requirement to maintain records of processing activities that, for example, must list all of the purposes for which personal data are being processed by an organisation (GDPR, Article 30, pp. 50–51).
- Obligations with regard to disclosing data to others, in particular where third parties are engaged to process personal data on behalf of a controller (GDPR, Article 28, pp. 49–50).

GDPR in a nutshell

In a nutshell, the GDPR is simple! It's a law that seeks to enable the free movement of data about individuals by: (a) providing a set of principles that should be observed when processing or considering processing personal data; (b) granting legal rights to individuals that enable them to enjoy their right to privacy and a private life; and (c) setting out obligations for those processing personal data to work within. In addition to that, the GDPR establishes a regulator, the ICO, and a series of penalties that may be applied to those who break the law.

Ensuring client confidentiality

Working within the framework of data protection law is more than just ensuring client confidentiality as, hopefully, is made clear above. Nonetheless, confidentiality is an essential feature of any patient-clinician relationship. But what is confidentiality? Confidentiality is one of the three features of 'security' and sits alongside integrity and availability. Other chapters of this book go into far more detail about security per se. The focus of this chapter is security as it relates to and is expressed in data protection legislation.

Before diving into confidentiality, we must briefly consider the concept of privacy by design and by default (PbD). This concept is contained within the GDPR (Article 25, p. 48) and requires systems of work, whether digital, computerised systems, or procedural, human behaviour-based systems, to be designed with privacy in mind. All processes and procedures that could impact privacy should be thought through and designed to embed privacy within them. And, furthermore, privacy should be the default setting. In truth we are some way from privacy by design and by default coursing through all of our organisations, but it will come. And it should not stop us from aspiring to adopt a PbD approach to the data-processing activities we ourselves are involved with. Everyone in an organisation should be taking a zero-tolerance approach to privacy. Risks should be identified and eliminated or reduced. Why should we tolerate inadequate data-processing arrangements that don't have PbD at their heart?

The systems of work that we use to process personal data, therefore, should be well thought out. And PbD is not a one-off exercise. Organisations need to foster a culture of continual improvement too. We need to accept that work-based systems can be reimagined and redesigned to improve efficiency and also privacy.

'Confidentiality' may have different meanings in different contexts but, in privacy law, it means 'keeping something secret or private'.

The sixth data protection principle of the GDPR requires that personal data is processed in a manner that ensures appropriate security of the personal data, including protection against unauthorised or unlawful processing and against accidental loss, destruction, or damage. It doesn't prescribe what it thinks is appropriate, unlike other standards, regulations, or laws, it leaves it up to us to determine that for ourselves. This approach means that we need to be mindful of the circumstances of many different use cases. What is appropriate security for one piece of information might not be appropriate for another. Or, what is appropriate security for one data subject might not be appropriate for a different one. However, with flexibility comes responsibility to think things through and get it right!

But the GDPR does set out what it is we are trying to protect data from. As discussed earlier in this chapter, the concept of lawful processing relates to the lawful bases and we need to ensure that we apply appropriate security measures to ensure that we don't subject any personal data to unlawful processing. For example, we need to guard against disclosing personal data to another organisation without a lawful basis, and from function creep of processing operations.

Given that the definition of processing is extremely broad, unauthorised processing is also very broadly framed. Unauthorised processing includes using personal data for purposes that have not been approved, as well as personal data being access by people who do not have the authority to access it. For example, disclosing personal data to people who are not authorised to have access to it would be a breach of security.

We also need to protect personal data from accidental (and malicious) loss, destruction, or damage. Most people can relate to lost laptops or files, and to ransomware or malware attacks that might damage or destroy information.

The security principle elaborates by setting out that we need to apply appropriate security by using appropriate technical and/or organisational measures. These technical measures might include anti-malware software or the encryption of data. Organisational measures might include training and awareness, policies and procedures, and compliance checks.

Data flows – it is not static

If we consider a typical data processing activity comprising the following steps, we can see that confidentiality might require a different approach at each step:

- Data collection/receipt
- Data storage
- Using/retrieving data
- Distributing data
- Creating data from data
- Disclosure of data
- Archiving of data
- End of life

Personal data might be received from other organisations or practitioners. Does it come with any overt conditions of use? Are these different from our established and standard terms of use? Do existing work systems and methods support these other conditions? Are you capable of storing such information in your data systems and apply more restricted access control, or restrict the use of the data, or the retention period?

You might also collect data using other methods. You might use paper forms in some circumstances. The paper form is simply the medium on which the data is recorded. What happens to it once the data is transcribed into another system such as a computer database? You might also collect personal data via recordings, scanning, or invasive medical procedures.

Knowing what you have and how you came by it is essential. It is also a useful exercise to trace and document data right through its lifecycle as this gives a baseline that can be analysed to seek efficiencies and improvements, as well as a baseline for future compliance-checking.

The GDPR tells us that we should ensure appropriate security is in place through implementing appropriate technical and organisational measures to ensure a level of security appropriate to the risks (GPDR, Articles 6(f), p. 36, and 32, pp. 51–52). It is useful sometime to think of risk not only in the context of risks to the rights and freedoms of individuals but also to the risk of non-compliance with the data protection law and other relevant matters such as professional codes of conduct. In that way we should be able to design and adopt good practices that are designed to ensure appropriate security in consideration of the risks in relevant dimensions.

Suggestions are made in the GDPR as to what we might consider implementing, such as pseudonymisation and anonymisation (GDPR, Article 32(1)(a), p. 51), but perhaps the most important are policies, procedures, and processes for regularly testing, assessing, and evaluating the effectiveness of technical and organisational measures implemented for ensuring the security of the processing. The timeframe for review differs from control to control. For example, some controls are monitored in real time by software systems such as file-integrity monitoring or intruder-detection systems. Other security measures might be checked daily through the review of logs. And it is not uncommon to conduct an annual disaster-recovery exercise. The point is that all measures should be reviewed on an appropriate timetable.

The final point to make about the GDPR's stance on security is that we are able to take into account the available technologies and other controls, and their cost, in relation to the nature, scope, context, and purposes of processing, and the risk of varying likelihood and severity for the rights and freedoms of people (GDPR, Article 32(1), p. 51). In practice this means that we must keep our controls under review as new technologies emerge and the cost of implementation falls. For example, there is no excuse for not applying full hard disk encryption to laptop computers, as the cost of implementation and impact on performance is negligible. We should think about data as an entity in its own right, detached from the systems used to process it, as the data may outlive the systems used to store and retrieve/distribute it. How are data transferred from an old system to a new one ensuring the data's integrity? What happens to the copies of the data on the old systems?

Summary

The essence of confidentiality for the purposes of this chapter is restricting access to and use of personal data. Other chapters address the 'how' of confidentiality. Some may even address a different take on the 'why'. The purpose of this chapter is to consider the data protection and privacy law and how elements of it relate to the topic. It aims to provide some insight into the legal framework in order to allow the medical practitioner and clinician to understand and apply the law confidently in their daily work. It aims to illustrate that the law in fact is flexibly worded and easy to work with. It has to be, as it was designed to regulate every industry and all types of personal data across the entirety of the EU. A final word of advice is this: If in doubt, reach out for assistance. You are not alone if you struggle to understand and work with the British data protection law.

References

BDSG (1977, 27 January). Federal Data Protection Act (1977). Law on Protection Against the Misuse of Personal Data in Data Processing. https://lawcat.berkeley.edu/record/465275?ln=en.

Computers and Personal Records Bill (1969). H.L. Deb 3 December 1969. *Hansard.* Vol. 306. https://hansard.parliament.uk/lords/1969-12-03/debates/60962194-ce0d-4f29-a252-15a19ee02840/ComputersAndPersonalRecords.

Convention for the Protection of Human Rights and Fundamental Freedoms (1950). Council of Europe Treaty Series 005, Council of Europe. https://rm.coe.int/1680a2353d.

Convention for the Protection of Individuals with regard to Automatic Processing of Personal Data (1980). European Treaty No. 108, 28 January 1980. https://rm.coe.int/1680078b37.

Data Protection Act (1984). Ch. 35. https://www.legislation.gov.uk/ukpga/1998/29/contents.

Data Protection Act (1998). Ch. 29. https://www.legislation.gov.uk/ukpga/1998/29/contents.

Data Protection Act (2018). Ch. 12. https://www.legislation.gov.uk/ukpga/2018/12/contents/enacted.

Data Surveillance Bill (1969). Deb 20 June 1969. *Hansard.* Vol. 785. https://hansard.parliament.uk/Commons/1969-06-20/debates/c79cee7f-6624-411e-8cf6-e1f7356ddba7/DataSurveillanceBill.

EC Directive (2003). The Privacy and Electronic Communications (EC Directive) Regulations 2003, UK Statutory Instruments 2003, No. 2426. https://www.legislation.gov.uk/uksi/2003/2426/contents/made.

EU Directive 95/46/EC (1995, 24 October). European Parliament and of the Council on the protection of individuals with regard to the processing of personal data and on the free movement of such data. OJ L281 pp. 31–50. https://eur-lex.europa.eu/legal-content/EN/TXT/?uri=OJ:L:1995:281:TOC.

EU Directive 2002/58/EC (2002, 12 July). European Parliament and the Council concerning the processing of personal data and the protection of privacy in the electronic communications sector (Directive on privacy and electronic communications). [2002] OJ L201, pp. 37–47. https://eur-lex.europa.eu/legal-content/EN/TXT/?uri=OJ:L:2002:201:TOC.

EU Directive 2009/136/EC (2009). European Parliament and the Council. [2009] OJ L337 pp. 11–36). https://eur-lex.europa.eu/legal-content/EN/TXT/?uri=OJ:L:2009:337:TOC.

EU Regulation 2016/679 (2016) Regulation 2016/679 of the European Parliament and of the Council of 27 April 2016 on the protection of natural persons with regard to the processing of personal data and on the free movement of such data [2016] (OJ L119 pp. 1–88). https://eur-lex.europa.eu/legal-content/EN/TXT/?uri=OJ:L:2016:119:TOC.

EU Directive 2016/680 (2016, 27 April). European Parliament and the Council on the protection of natural persons with regard to the processing of personal data by competent authorities for the purposes of the prevention, investigation, detection or prosecution of criminal offences or the execution of criminal penalties, and on the free movement of such data. [2016] OJ L119 pp. 89–131. https://eur-lex.europa.eu/legal-content/EN/TXT/?uri=celex%3A32016L0680.

GSA https://www.gsa.gov/directive/gsa-rules-of-behavior-for-handling-personally-identifiable-information

Law Post Office (Revenues) Act (1710). 9 Anne c.10, 25 November 1710. https://www.gbps.org.uk/information/sources/acts/1710-11-25_Act-9-Anne-cap-10.php.

OECD (1980). Guidelines governing the protection of privacy and transborder flow of personal data. 23 September 1980. https://www.oecd-ilibrary.org/science-and-technology/oecd-guidelines-on-the-protection-of-privacy-and-transborder-flows-of-personal-data_9789264196391-en.

Official Secrets Act (1898). 52 & 53 Victoria, c.52. https://statutes.org.uk/site/the-statutes/nineteenth-century/1889-52-53-victoria-c-52-official-secrets-act/.

Report of Committee on Privacy (1972). Cmnd. 5012. HMSO.

Report of the Committee on Data Protection (1978). HMSO.

Right of Privacy Bill (1961) [H.L.] HL Deb 13 March 1961. *Hansard.* Vol. 229, cc607–661, paras 2–6. https://api.parliament.uk/historic-hansard/lords/1961/mar/13/right-of-privacy-bill-hl.

Warren, S.D., & Brandeis, L.D. (1890, 15 December). The right to privacy. *Harvard Law Review, 4,* 193–220. https://www.cs.cornell.edu/~shmat/courses/cs5436/warren-brandeis.pdf.

4 Privacy rights and freedoms

Rowenna Fielding

This chapter examines the nature of privacy from a social, legal, and psychological perspective. By offering examples and references, I hope to assist the psychology professional, you, in recognising and adopting measures to protect privacy; for your clients, your peers and yourselves.

What is privacy?

- A legal right?
- A social strategy?
- A psychological necessity?
- A sense, feeling or experience?

All these descriptions are accurate, yet none of them is complete. So, what is privacy?

To study privacy is to delve into the complexities of human interpersonal relationships, our collective and individual needs, our evolving cultural mores, and technological capabilities. 'Privacy' means different things to different people, depending on context and circumstances. Ask a lawyer, a software developer, and a philosopher to define privacy; the answer will be different each time. To the lawyer, privacy concerns legislation, rights, and precedence. For the software developer, privacy is a question of configuration, technical settings, and choice of architecture. A philosopher might view privacy in terms of moral relativity and ethics, or metaphysical theories of consciousness. One of the most (entertaining/annoying – delete as appropriate) aspects of privacy is that it's such a big, shape-shifting, fuzzy monster of a topic. Just to make things even more complicated, privacy comes in a variety of flavours, including:

- **Interactional privacy**, which relates to quantity and quality of interactions with others (Burgoon et al, 1989; Laufer & Wolfe, 1977).
- **Territorial or physical privacy**, which relates to personal space and being touched by others (Klopfer & Rubenstein, 1977).
- **Expressive privacy**, regarding expression of one's self or identity (DeCew, 1997).
- **Psychological privacy**, concerning one's thoughts, emotions and the revelation of them (Burgoon et al., 1989; Stuart et al., 2019).

DOI: 10.4324/9781003364184-5

And perhaps the most widely recognised version in the age of 'big data':

- **Informational [or data] privacy**, relating to an individual's right to control the degree to which information about them is communicated (Westin, 1967).

'Privacy' is evidently easier to describe than it is to define. Thankfully, it is not necessary to provide incontrovertible mathematical proofs for any dimension of privacy in order to understand its significance or adopt practices that uphold it.

For the purposes of this chapter – to provide a foundational understanding of the nature of privacy and some solid, actionable intelligence with which to go about upholding it – the most helpful working definition of privacy is this one:

> Selective control over interactions between self (or one's group) and others, the ultimate aim of which is to enhance autonomy and/or to minimise vulnerability.
> (orig. Margulis, 1977)

Why is privacy necessary?

Limits On Power

protection limits the power that others can wield over us, by allowing us to set boundaries on how and when we can be observed, engaged with or influenced.

Privacy is a defensive shield for other rights and freedoms that are necessary for maintaining an equitable balance of powers; such as freedom of conscience and belief, freedom of association and movement, or freedom of speech and expression. Protection of these freedoms is critical to participatory democracy and functional justice systems.

Privacy protects the presumption of innocence – in affording an accused person the benefit of the doubt, the state is required to present evidence that they were in fact up to no good. If there were no right to privacy, it could easily be assumed that an accused's reluctance to disclose the intimate details of their every thought and act were an indication of dishonesty. The burden of proof would be reversed, and innocence would be even harder to defend than it already is.

The social contract

Privacy allows individuals to develop unique personalities while participating in social units, balancing the benefits of individual thinking with the advantages of coordinated group action. If all of the members of a group are obliged to think, behave, and act alike, then that group will be less resilient to change or disruption than if its members are permitted to diversify. Denial of privacy is a common feature of authoritarian regimes, based on the theory that if no one is allowed their own personal space, then they'll have minimal opportunities for sedition.

Dignity and safety

One cannot treat an individual with respect unless their privacy boundaries are also respected. Allowing time and space for others to form their own ideas and make their own decisions, trusting that they will make good choices, is a critical ingredient for healthy, functional relationships. Constantly observing, judging, intervening with, or manipulating another person sends them the message that they are not trusted, or considered capable enough to be let alone – or that their interests and preferences simply don't matter. Many abusive domestic relationships feature some form of privacy denial, or asymmetry, as a tactic for coercion and psychological control.

The right to privacy

At various points in history, societies and individuals have recognised privacy as a natural, or moral right that is necessary for the wellbeing of individuals and for general social harmony; but, in everyday discourse, privacy rights are most commonly spoken of in terms of legal rights; e.g. as claims or entitlements that are defined and can be secured by the application of legal process.

When human rights were formally established in 1948 (Universal Declaration of Human Rights, or UDHR), privacy was explicitly mentioned (albeit without much detail): 'No one shall be subjected to arbitrary interference with [their] privacy, family, home, or correspondence, nor to attacks upon [their] honour and reputation. Everyone has the right to the protection of the law against such interference or attacks' (UDHR, 1948).

Article 12, Universal Declaration of Human Rights

The Universal Declaration of Human Rights was created in the hope that the massacres and other atrocities committed by various states (*not just the Nazis*) could be avoided in future by recognition of what it means to be human and by the acknowledgement of human needs.

> Whereas recognition of the inherent dignity and of the equal and inalienable rights of all members of the human family is the foundation of freedom, justice and peace in the world,
>
> Whereas disregard and contempt for human rights have resulted in barbarous acts which have outraged the conscience of mankind, and the advent of a world in which human beings shall enjoy freedom of speech and belief and freedom from fear and want has been proclaimed as the highest aspiration of the common people,
>
> Whereas it is essential, if man is not to be compelled to have recourse, as a last resort, to rebellion against tyranny and oppression, that human rights should be protected by the rule of law.
>
> (UDHR, 1948)

The UDHR was later officially translated into law by the passing of the International Bill of Human Rights and subsequent treaties were made between nations. However, the degree to which privacy rights are established and protected in domestic law varies wildly between cultures and jurisdictions. Some nations have yet to establish any privacy legislation at all, while others have chosen to address privacy within specific domains, such as healthcare (USA: Health Insurance Portability and Accountability Act 1996), credit scoring (Chile: Ley No. 21.398 – D.Oficial 24/12/2021; *Spanish text only*), online communications (EU: Directive 2002/58/EC, the 'ePrivacy Directive'), or federal government (Canada: Privacy Act, RSC, 1985, c. P-21).

Privacy is seldom an absolute right. Where they exist in law, privacy rights are 'qualified' rights, meaning that they can be selectively overridden if doing so is necessary for protection of other social interests. For example:

- Your right to physical privacy is suspended when a police officer carries out a lawful search of your person – they can touch you without your permission to detect or prevent a criminal act.
- Your medical privacy rights to refuse treatment or to confidentiality of your records may be set aside if you're infected with a dangerous and highly contagious pathogen.
- Any or all of your privacy rights may be overridden by the interests of national security, if you are suspected or convicted of being a terrorist or an espionage agent.

As you can see, there's a lot of 'it depends' involved in privacy law. The right to privacy is an inalienable fundamental human rights, but exactly what that looks like varies from place to place.

Privacy myth-busting

Having established what privacy *is*, let us turn for a moment to the question of what privacy *isn't*. As a privacy and data protection professional, I frequently encounter myths, misinformation, and muddles about privacy that have taken root (as a result of poor-quality journalism and substandard corporate training) and keep propagating. Privacy myths derail well-intentioned efforts, resulting in unnecessary costs for organisations and potential exposure to privacy harms for people.

Privacy does not mean isolation

Isolation is an absence of interaction with others, whether through choice (self-isolation), through circumstance, or through rejection by others. If a person were to assert extreme boundaries in the name of privacy, they may cause themselves to become isolated; however, privacy and isolation are essentially divergent goals – privacy helps individuals to integrate within social units without sacrificing their uniqueness, whereas an isolated person is more of an anti-social unit.

Privacy does not mean the opposite of 'in public'

It's just not that simple.

For example, imagine a person reading alone in a public library. While they are 'out in public' in the sense that anyone could come into the library and observe them, they still have plenty of privacy as long as no one gets too close or tries to interfere with them.

Privacy cannot be switched 'on' or 'off'

Privacy isn't a binary switch that changes a state of 'no boundaries at all' to 'complete seclusion' (or vice versa).

This characterisation of privacy as an 'all or nothing' zero-sum proposition is absurdly reductionist, and one that casts doubt on the good faith of its proponents. It is commonly expressed as a false dichotomy between 'privacy vs safety' or 'privacy vs free online content'. To subscribe to this view is to ignore the infinities of nuance and context that govern human interpersonal relationships.

- You can welcome a close friend's candid opinion of your outfit while expecting random strangers to refrain from offering unsolicited criticism of your style choices.
- You could expect gratitude for grabbing someone's arm to pull them out of the path of an out-of-control vehicle, but you wouldn't be thanked for yanking someone out of your way so you can jump a queue.
- You take your clothes off to prepare for a full-body spa massage, but that wouldn't be appropriate for a pedicure.
- You're not obliged to inform your boss about the fan fiction you write under a pseudonym during your leisure time.

Context matters. In fact, when it comes to privacy, **context is everything**.

Privacy does not mean concealment

Rejecting or evading scrutiny and interference is a tactic which can be employed to preserve one's privacy (legitimately or otherwise), but the tactic is not 'privacy' in and of itself.

For example, a person might obscure the details of their Internet activities from government, commercial, or criminal snooping by using a virtual private network (VPN), but if they post and browse under their 'real' (i.e. state-registered) name, then concealment of their online traffic won't protect them from state surveillance or commercial profiling.

Privacy does not mean secrecy

As with concealment, secrecy may be used to protect a person's privacy, but neither the act nor the method of keeping something secret is necessarily related to privacy as an objective.

For example, a corporation may keep the nature of its best-selling formula a secret out of concern for its market advantage. Corporations may rely on confidentiality, but they can't have 'privacy' for themselves because privacy is only for humans.

Privacy does not mean data protection

Data protection is often confused with privacy because the two topics are closely related. Data protection is a set of rules and requirements established in law for protecting the rights and freedoms of individuals (of which privacy is only one, there are many others) when personal data relating to them is processed, so that organisations can get useful stuff done with data in non-abusive ways.

Although they intersect in many ways, privacy is bigger than data protection – and data protection is bigger than privacy.

Privacy does not mean information security

Another pair of different-but-intersecting topics that are frequently confused with each other – information security is the practice of protecting the confidentiality, integrity, and availability of information assets relative to risk. It is possible to implement robust information security while neglecting or infringing privacy; and privacy can nonetheless be upheld in an environment where no information assets exist.

Privacy does not mean mandatory consent

Consent is a mechanism for formalising relationship parameters that can serve the purpose of privacy, but does not fulfil that purpose by itself. Reliance on consent can actually undermine privacy objectives, if the process is mishandled or the tactic is misapplied.

- If the other person
    - has no power to refuse or prevent the interaction,
    - if they are coerced, manipulated or deceived,
    - if they cannot change their mind later on, *or*
    - if they don't understand what they're agreeing to

- then relying on their consent to interact (which includes access or use of information relating to them) is an ethically dubious practice, and likely to be legally questionable.

Your mortgage adviser should not gossip about your appearance, the tidiness of your household, or the state of your marriage, because those topics are simply none of their business. Asking for your consent to gossip about you would not protect your privacy in this scenario – those subjects should simply be off limits as a matter of courtesy (and common sense).

Sometimes a person doesn't – or shouldn't – have a choice about whether to assert a privacy boundary, particularly if declining to give consent may put themselves or others at imminent risk of harm.

For example, employees at a nuclear power station would not be expected to give (or permitted to refuse) their consent to carry personal radiation monitors. As a radiation leak could threaten the health or lives of all the workers (and potentially anyone else who lives nearby), the collective need for identification of rogue radioactivity outweighs the individual's preference not to be monitored.

Privacy paradigms

Back in the 'days of yore', before the combustion engine and electronic communications, privacy controls were mostly a matter of physical separation – putting distance, barrier materials (such as clothing, walls, shutters, etc.), or social protocols between bodies to indicate that certain interactions would be undesirable. To keep a person under covert surveillance, or meddle in their affairs without them noticing, would be difficult and require considerable resources.

Zip forward a few hundred years, to where advances in communications and travel technology had produced widespread literacy, mass printing, public transport, the telegraph, and the telephone. People could now interact in greater numbers, at greater speeds and with less effort. Self-separation was still mostly based on physical distancing, physical barriers, and social protocol, but the degree of effort required to maintain that separation was increased. As links between people became denser, the resources needed to negate separation efforts diminished relative to the common means. One-to-many communications mechanisms, such as the printing press, or the telephone party line, allowed interactions to occur in greater numbers, with greater ease, outside the limitations of physical presence. Incidents of observation and intervention were more difficult to detect amid the background noise of tech-extended social interactions.

And then – computers happened.

With the advent of data, automation, and high-speed digital communications technology, observation and influence were no longer restricted by physical distance, or the limits of human physiology. Information could be obtained, instructions sent, messages received at the speed of electricity. Hundreds, thousands, millions of people could be interacted with simultaneously – and below their perception thresholds – by manipulation of data. Among all of this capability and complexity, the effort and rewards of maintaining respect for people's privacy boundaries have respectively bloated and shrivelled, yet the protections that privacy affords are more greatly needed than at any other time in human history.

Digital privacy

As with every technology humanity has ever developed, the rush to make use of all the shiny new possibilities, left wider implications such as safety and the potential for adverse consequences by the wayside. As Dr Ian Malcolm famously states in

Jurassic Park: 'Your scientists were so preoccupied with whether they could, they didn't stop to think if they should.' There is no better summary of the disgraceful neglect – or even outright hostility – with which digital privacy has been treated in the digital marketplace thus far.

Digital privacy is the same as any other flavour of privacy – it is your moral and legal right to make your own choices (within reason), to be free from observation and interference (within reason), to protect your other rights and freedoms (within reason), and to be as much the master of your own self as you care to be (within reason).

However, digital privacy is much more challenging to uphold and maintain, not least due to the sheer volume and scale of digital interactions that are conducted each minute as well as the global distribution of digital economies. These factors make maintaining digital privacy difficult enough on their own, even without the presence of entire industries that exist explicitly to 'datafy' and commoditise every aspect of human existence. It is these, more than any individual tycoon, dictator, or aggrieved member of the public, that represent the greatest threat to privacy in the digital arena.

Surveillance advertising

The majority of electronic devices you encounter in day-to-day living will be generating data about you, and mostly likely sending that data elsewhere to be categorised, analysed, and put to use. Electronic surveillance is now ubiquitous and inescapable – you may choose not to have a smartphone, but you can't stop other people's smartphones from registering your presence. You can decline to install a smart speaker or smart TV in your home, reject the robot vacuum cleaner, refuse Internet-connected fridges, coffeemakers, toasters, ovens, and toilets, drive an older model of car without onboard computers, do all your shopping in person – but your bank will still be monitoring and profiling your purchasing habits, there will still be commercially and personally owned cameras capturing your image wherever you go, and every move you make online will still be tracked and used to generate inferences about what you might be persuaded to buy, amplify, support, or vote for.

Targeted advertising is currently the Internet's dominant economic model – even software and services that require payment to use are nonetheless vectors for harvesting information about their users. With the use of tracking technologies, such as cookies, web beacons, and fingerprinting, detailed profiles can be built of any person's lifestyle, financial situation, and character, which are then used for real-time programmatic advertising (an online auction system that uses algorithms to match advertisements with Internet users in the seconds it takes to load a webpage).

Imagine a world in which almost every aspect of your existence can be observed, scrutinised, judged, labelled, nudged, and exploited by unseen persons, at the touch of a button, without your participation or even your awareness; and all without a moment's consideration of your rights or your welfare.

You live in that world right now.

> [C]ompanies personalise products, processes and advertisement by approximat-
> ing and predicting customer attributes and behaviours through profiling and data
> analysis. Companies collect the necessary input data for these operations through
> various methods. In addition to requesting information or observing offline
> behaviour, they collect data by logging and tracking user activities; by scraping,
> sharing, and trading data; as well as by merging or acquiring companies.
> Researchers have identified multiple fields of application that rely on tracking and
> profiling; these include marketing, customer analytics, credit scoring and perso-
> nal finance, fraud prevention and risk management, employee monitoring, hiring
> and workforce analytics, insurance, healthcare, and e-learning.
>
> (European Parliamentary Research Service Report, December 2022)

Tracking technologies

To understand and protect digital privacy, you need to know a bit about how it
works. The following section describes the most prevalent types of digital tracking
in non-technical terms.

Cookies

A cookie, as you will have no doubt been informed by various online pop-ups and
policies, is a text file that tags your browser client (the program you use for looking at web pages on the Internet) with a unique identifier so that web servers can
recognise it. The text file can also contain other data that gives the web server
information about how to interact with your browser.

A cookie is like a digital label displaying a unique name in computer language
that sticks to your computer/phone/etc. until its expiry date is reached or you
remove it by deleting the text file.

How cookies work

Cookies work by keeping track of your browser's 'conversations' with Internet servers.

1 You connect to a web server.
2 That server checks to see if your device is wearing any cookies that it can read,
  and sends the cookies that it needs to use (along with any that you may have
  given consent for) into your browser's storage. This is called 'setting' the
  cookie and it means sending instructions to your browser to create the text
  files and put certain information into them.
3 If there are already cookies present that the server can access, then the server
  may send updated information to them.
4 The information from the cookie text is used by the web server to do something (whatever job the cookie has been put there for).

There are lots of reasons why your browser needs to be uniquely recognisable to web servers. For example:

- Allowing conversations between your browser and web servers to continue if they are interrupted.
- Sharing the job of sending web content to your browser across multiple servers (for speed/reliability) and make it arrive in the right place and in the right order.

Cookies also enable convenient features, such as the facility to remember your preference settings on a particular site.

Most of these uses of cookies are not a threat to privacy per se, provided that appropriate security settings have been put in place to prevent the cookies being tinkered with by unauthorised persons. However, the other uses are the principal reason for cookies gaining such a bad reputation among Internet users, as they facilitate mass surveillance, profiling, and targeting of interactions with little regard for the 'right to be let alone'.

- Identifying devices used by the same user, when and where they are used to build a more complete picture of that person's activities.
- Allowing tracking online activity across huge networks in order to make inferences and statistical guesses about people's characteristics.
- Using profiles developed from tracking and inference to target, curate, conceal, and influence a person's online (and offline) experiences.

Web beacons, aka tracking pixels

A 'web beacon' (or 'bug') is an invisible image, usually 1x1 pixel in size, which is used to track interactions with webpages, emails, and app screens. Digital marketers use these tracking pixels to monitor the effectiveness of their campaigns, and cause adverts to 'follow' website visitors when they move on to other sites. The most basic version of a tracking pixel works like this:

1   You open an email, or land on a webpage.
2   The email or website page contains scripting code (a form of mini-program) that calls out to a remote server where the image is stored.
3   The remote server logs the call and supplies the image, which is loaded as part of the email or webpage. It's invisible to human eyes because it's so small.
4   By analysing the data that comes from the 'call' to the remote server, the following information can be obtained about the person who opened the email or webpage:
    - what data and time they looked at the email or page
    - their approximate location (from the IP address of the connection)
    - the make and model of device they are using

- the operating system of the device
- the email or browser client that the pixel has been loaded by
- the screen resolution of the device.

Tracking and analysis of the results is done by algorithm, as there aren't enough hours in the day for human beings to go through the enormous amounts of data that these tracking technologies generate.

Fingerprinting

This is a method of using information that can be obtained remotely about your device or your browser, to identify a 'fingerprint'. Since no two devices are likely to have exactly the same combinations of software and settings, browser fingerprinting is a highly accurate way of distinguishing and tracking unique Internet users.

Advertising identifier

A unique number assigned to a device (usually a smartphone or tablet), which is used to deliver and track digital ads displayed on the device. The AD-ID gets passed along to servers through cookies and tracking pixels.

None of these technologies are inherently 'bad', but their use for surveillance, profiling, and automated judgement do pose a threat to your, and everyone else's, privacy. Although many jurisdictions have laws in place to limit unfair or harmful uses of these technologies and the data they produce, compliance with those laws is generally viewed as burden to be minimised, rather than a protective legal or social obligation.

Data harms

'Data harms' are adverse consequences for people that have arisen through careless use of digital tracking, profiling, and automated decision-making technologies. Apart from those obvious and direct harms, such as the deliberate misuse of confidential information leading to injury or distress, many data harms (such as discrimination and exploitation) are produced by stochastic processes, meaning that although certain types of adverse consequence can be foreseen, it is impossible to predict exactly when, where, and to whom.

The most significant and likely form of data harms that your clients could be exposed to are the consequences of a confidentiality breach, and discrimination caused by digital tracking in tools and systems that you rely on for your work. Even if you scrupulously observe client confidentiality and data security obligations when interacting with other people, you also need to keep a sharp eye on the digital interactions that your work incurs, to prevent them from 'outing' your clients.

But how could that happen? Well, it probably goes something like this:

1   You have a web or social media presence for advertising your services, and for engaging with clients. Unless you have conducted a thorough review of digital privacy protections around this presence (whether it is a website or a social media account), it is highly likely that there will be a significant amount of digital tracking built into the platform and tools you use to manage it. These features will either be included and enabled by default, or you will have been encouraged to make use of them to 'maximise engagement' or 'improve your marketing/search engine optimisation metrics'.

2   A client, or relative of a client engages with your online presence – perhaps to make an enquiry, or to look up your contact details for later reference.

3   The digital tracking mechanisms described above log and feed the client's information (identifiers, activities logged) to advertising networks to be appended to data profiles relating to that person or device.

4   That information is then used to curate and mediate the client's (or prospective client's) online experience – from the advertisements they are shown to the content automatically recommended or made available to them.

A forensic report conducted by Cracked Labs (2022) revealed that gambling companies target gambling ads at people who have been profiled through digital tracking as gambling addicts. Although there is a wealth of evidence to support the harmful effects of surveillance advertising, and the discriminatory effects of data profiling, regulation of these activities is still at a very early stage.

This is not some paranoid science fiction dystopia. This is the reality of how surveillance advertising and the attention economy is designed to function.

Concerns about uses of data from digital tracking and profiling in automated risk assessment have also been identified in areas such as employment, housing, financial services, and social care. Whether or not the inferences made about a person based on their online activity are accurate, making covert inferences about a person's mental or physical health in order to judge their value, or suitability, or risk, is a practice fraught with potential for harms.

In addition to the intentional effects of data profiling, the unintended consequences resulting of mass data harvesting and digital profiling also give rise to concerns about digital privacy. In 2016, a psychiatrist in the US was notified by patients that they had begun to receive 'friend' recommendations for each other's Facebook accounts. How could this happen? Due to Facebook's secrecy around its data operations, there is no way to be certain. There are a number of ways in which each patient's digital data trails could have been correlated with those of other patients, such as:

- Through location tracking on patients' smartphones or fitness trackers, logging visits to the psychiatrist's place of practice.
- By upload of the psychiatrist's (and/or patients') contacts information to Facebook's servers (by installation of WhatsApp or Facebook Messenger), and identification of 'mutuals' in the listed contact numbers.

'Smart' devices also pose a threat to confidentiality, especially those with audio or video recording features. Sound and video files may be retrieved by the device manufacturer and analysed to improve voice and image recognition quality, or to obtain insights that can assist with targeted advertising. In some reported cases, smart devices have erroneously sent copies of recordings to third parties

Privacy in practice

It would be an exaggeration (and defeatist!) to claim that there is 'no privacy' in digital or that 'privacy is dead'. True, most digital products and services were developed without regard to privacy (at best), or with the very intention of thoroughly infringing it (at worst). Also true, maintaining boundaries around your rights and dignity is challenging, not least because of the sheer volume and scale of possible interactions that 'digital' permits. It might be tempting to let it all slide, to shrug and conclude that any effort to protect privacy boundaries is doomed and therefore not worth attempting. This is not true – and wouldn't be an acceptable professional position, even if it were.

The relationship between practitioner and client is covered by a professional and legal duty of confidence. However, unless you are careful to protect digital privacy boundaries around yourself and your clients, the fact, if not the nature, of your client relationships may be disclosed to thousands of companies around the world. Whether or not that information is used in ways that cause discernible harms to those individuals is moot: the data should not be exposed to third parties who have no legitimate need to know as a result of action or inaction by a mental health professional.

How to protect your clients' privacy

- Comply with data protection and electronic privacy laws that apply in your location.
- Disable or physically remove all smart devices and voice assistant functions when conducting client sessions.
- Do not use free or consumer-market tools or services to store, transmit, or analyse information relating to clients, whether or not you believe the individuals may be identifiable from that information.
- You should only use software and services for your work activities under commercial licenses (never 'free for personal use' or ad-funded). This especially applies to any tool, platform, or service for video conferencing, note-taking or record-keeping, calendar-scheduling, and correspondence
- Scrutinise the privacy information for any service you use. If the privacy notice indicates that usage data may be used for marketing and advertising purposes, there is a high risk that using that tool or service would undermine your clients' privacy. This includes payment processing, business administration, and personal organisation services.

If you have a separate phone handset for work

- Turn off collection of performance analytics and advertising data in all device and app settings.
- Don't install any messaging apps on that handset unless you are confident that they have been specifically evaluated for strength of confidentiality and approved for use within a healthcare context.
- Don't install any games, media, shopping, or news apps on that device. Delete default apps that you will not use for work purposes.
- Turn off location tracking.
- Turn off collection of performance analytics and advertising data in all device and app settings.
- Only engage verified professionals to perform technical support work on the device, and only with a formal IT services contract in place that meets data protection standards for your locale.

If you don't use a separate phone for work

You should:

- Obtain and start using one if at all possible.

Otherwise:

- Avoid using the 'contacts list' on your personal smartphone to store client contact information. If a second phone handset is not feasible, then client information should be kept within a separate app or document.
- Delete client information from call and message logs right away.
- Avoid making, storing, or accessing recordings of client sessions or client notes on your personal phone. If you must access files stored in the Cloud (professional-grade platforms only, no free or data-paid services), make sure that synchronising and caching features are disabled so that they do not remain on your personal phone when not in use.
- Disable WiFi, Bluetooth, and location tracking functions when you leave your home and/or office.

If you recommend or encourage the use of apps for meditation, mood journaling, or other supportive activities, try to avoid recommending apps that harvest data for advertising. This information should be in the app's privacy notice. If no privacy information is supplied, the app is probably not safe for the client to use.

If you have a website

- Use only professional hosting services; avoid free platforms as they will not provide adequate levels of privacy, security, or technical support.

- Use a tool such as webbkoll.dataskydd.net/ or privacyscore.org to identify potential privacy problems; or engage a privacy professional to conduct a review of the site's configuration.
- If you outsource your website's design to a third party, make sure that your contract with them clearly specifies:

  ○ The provider shall be familiar with the requirements of data protection and e-privacy laws that are relevant to the purpose and configuration of the site.
  ○ The site shall be designed, built, and maintained in compliance with those requirements, which should include comprehensive documentation of all functions and dataflows, which should be made available to you.

- If your website features an enquiry form, check whether submitted form data is saved to the web server (and, if so, clear it out regularly), and/or if it is transmitted to third parties (you must have a contract with them that clearly specifies the high confidentiality level of that data).
- Arrange for any inbuilt advertising or social media tracking pixels, widgets, or scripts to be disabled or removed.
- Only use privacy-safe analytics tools (such as Matomo/PiWik or Plausible) to track visitors to your site.

If you've made it this far, you will hopefully now have a clearer understanding of what 'privacy' is, what it is for, and why it's important to pay attention to it – especially in the age of 'big digital'.

References

Burgoon, J., Parrott, R., Poire, B., Kelley, D., Walther, J., & Perry, D. (1989). Maintaining and restoring privacy through communication in different types of relationships. *Journal of Social and Personal Relationships, 6,* 131-158. https://doi.org/10.1177/026540758900600201.

Cracked Labs (2022). Digital profiling in the online gambling industry. https://crackedlabs.org/en/gambling-data.

DeCew, J. (1997). Privacy and information technology. *Center for the Study of Ethics in Society Papers, 10*(2). https://scholarworks.wmich.edu/ethics_papers/40.

European Parliamentary Research Service Report (December 2022). Unpacking 'commercial surveillance': The state of tracking. https://www.europarl.europa.eu/RegData/etudes/BRIE/2022/739266/EPRS_BRI(2022)739266_EN.pdf.

Klopfer, P.H., & Rubenstein, D.I. (1977). The concept privacy and its biological basis. *Journal of Social Issues, 33,* 52-65. https://doi.org/10.1111/j.1540-4560.1977.tb01882.x.

Laufer, R.S., & Wolfe, M. (1977). Privacy as a concept and a social issue: A multidimensional developmental theory. *Journal of Social Issues, 33*(3), 22-42. https://doi.org/10.1111/j.1540-4560.1977.tb01880.x.

Margulis, S.T. (1977). Conceptions of privacy: Current status and next steps. *Journal of Social Issues*, *33*(*3*), 5-21. https://doi.org/10.1111/j.1540-4560.1977.tb01879.x.

Stuart, A., Bandara, A.K., & Levine, M. (2019). The psychology of privacy in the digital age. *Social and Personality Psychology Compass*, *13*(*11*), e12507. https://doi.org/10.1111/spc3.12507.

UDHR (1948). https://www.un.org/en/about-us/universal-declaration-of-human-rights.

Westin, Alan F. (1967). *Privacy and Freedom*. New York: Atheneum, 196-197.

5 Why cybersecurity matters and why training is essential

Cameron Broadbent and Melanie Oldham

Why cybersecurity matters

You've probably come into this book thinking you're not a worthwhile target for cybercriminals. The information you hold on yourself and those in your care doesn't have any value, right? What's the worst thing that could really happen if it fell into the wrong hands?

These are some of the most common misconceptions people have about personal information. Just because you can't conceptualise a way of utilising information doesn't mean that other people can't. When those other people are professional criminals you can certainly believe they know a way to make use of every scrap of personal information they can harvest.

The value of personal information

It's easy to underestimate the value of personal information. The privacy paradox (Barth & De Jong, 2017) found that, whilst people may claim to be concerned about privacy and personal data, they are very unlikely to take any action to prevent or protect the disclosure of their personal data. First, I want to show you what makes personal information so valuable to cybercriminals, especially when that information is sensitive. I'm not talking about bank details here, but about traumas from a vulnerable person's past being used against them.

Search online for the Vastaamo Psychotherapy Service (Finlex, 2021). You will find several stories of patients who had their information stolen from the company, and who then had it held against them for ransom.

Ralston (2021) reported how one of the victims, Jere, was attacked. Jere went to the centre when he was a teenager. While there he spoke about his abusive parents, self-harm, and thoughts of ending his life. What Jere didn't know was that his therapist was typing this information up onto Vestaamo's servers after their sessions.

Some years later, Jere received a ransom demand after a breach of the Vastaamo Psychotherapy Service. He received an email containing his personal details and the centre he attended. The message was simple: if he did not pay the ransom, all the information he had disclosed to the therapist would be posted online for the world to see. Friends, family, potential employers, and anyone else would be able to see it.

DOI: 10.4324/9781003364184-6

The ransom demanded was €200 within 24 hours, or €500 within 48 hours. It might not sound like the amount would have been worth the effort of breaching the company, but imagine this being multiplied across the thousands of patients who had their information stolen. Just because you aren't recording people's financial information doesn't mean it's worthless.

Now consider someone in your care believing that they are in a space where they can talk freely and openly, only for that trust to be betrayed and their information used against them in a cyber-related attack? How would that affect a person's view of you, your profession, and your institution? Would they ever truly open themselves up again, through fear of something similar happening a second time?

This story shows you just one of the many ways in which cybercriminals can use the sensitive information that you record of people in your care. Stories like this show why you must treat the information you have recorded about people with the utmost care, and as securely as possible.

Attacks aren't restricted to banks and businesses, they can be on public institutions and individuals as well. As more of our lives are lived online, more of each of us is becoming personal data. 'We are in the middle of a "personal data gold rush" driven by the dominance of advertising as the primary source of revenue for most online companies' (Chaudhry et al., 2015, p. 1).

Personal information does not need to be used directly against the owner for it to be damaging either. Armour (2022) reported that when the Scottish Association of Mental Health was breached, the result was 12 GB of data held on patients going up for sale on the dark web, an area of the Internet often associated with illegal activities, such as drug trafficking, weapons sales, and other criminal enterprises.

In the aftermath of this attack, the Scottish Association of Mental Health decided that a full review of the information technology (IT) system and daily practices should be performed. Changes were made and the security of the association saw major improvement.

The problem is the cost it took to convince them that security was something they needed to be concerned about. It took losing personal and sensitive information. The cost of negligence is so often paid by those most innocent.

To give you an idea of just how much information 12 GB is, you would need about 100,000 emails or 64,782 pages of Microsoft Word documents. All that data went up for sale on the dark web. How far this damage stretched, we do not know.

So, what do cybercriminals do with information they purchase? There are several different uses, beyond holding the victims to ransom. Identity fraud and spear-phishing (see below) are just two more examples of attack vectors that are growing every year.

Spear-phishing is a targeted form of phishing email that is specifically designed for an individual or small group. 'These attacks are more targeted than phishing emails and use personal information about their intended victims in an attempt to seem authentic and improve the likelihood that the target responds to the attacks' (Halevi et al., 2015, p. 1).

You can imagine how valuable the sensitive information gathered by the Scottish Association of Mental Health would be in this context. Being able to include National Insurance numbers, or purporting to be from legitimate people that the victims would expect to receive emails or phone calls from would be deadly.

Identity fraud is another reason why someone would buy personal information on the dark web. It is not only possible to create accounts with banks for loans or credit card companies, but, for example, supermarkets and retailers offer store cards that allow a person to purchase items from them.

Even if a person is not necessarily wealthy, their identity is still valuable. For example, known criminals who cannot move freely on their own identity find great value in stolen ones.

The personal information of all people has value to some extent. To be put in the privileged position of having access to other people's information requires you to operate in a way that helps to protect what they have entrusted to you.

'The collaborative relationship that develops between therapist and patient, referred to as the therapeutic alliance, is a key component of mental health care' (Cromer et al., 2017, p. 520).

When a person is put in a position of trust by another, the damage done by not operating daily practices in a safe and secure way and breaking that trust is exponentially greater when the information confided is an individual's most sensitive and personal information.

Physical data

Many people think that data only counts if the data are digital, but this is not the case. Information you write down on notepads and paper is looked at in the same way within security. This is because the information is still personal, sensitive, and can be exploited.

People can make the mistake of thinking that, if it's in a notepad no one can get hold of it. They don't consider the possibility of losing the notepad or of the bag holding the notepad being stolen.

There is a bond of trust between the person who is giving sensitive information and the person who receives it. This is not simply for patients and carers but for anyone who gives personal information. Would you have an expectation that information you provide someone is treated with care and safeguarded as best as possible?

Imagine how you would feel if you had gone to someone to speak openly about a difficult experience. They write down what you say and leave the notepad out in the office for all to see, or they lose it, or it is stolen. Would you think, oh it doesn't really matter, because it isn't your bank details, or would you feel concerned, angry, and let down?

Why you are a target

Those working in social care are targeted by cybercriminals more than you might think. From their research, Aldawood and Skinner (2019, p. 73) found that

'Awareness campaigns for employees should supersede the individual bias and eliminate thoughts that such attacks "will not happen to me"'.

It's vital that your training works towards changing this notion, because those in social care don't just have access to a lot of information, it's also very sensitive. Should you think of yourself as not worth attacking, you will make yourself into the perfect target.

Muncaster (2022) reported on a cyberattack on Hackney Council, London, UK, that happened in October 2020: the Council was forced to spend £12 million recovering from it. The breach impacted various branches of the organisation, including social care and housing registers.

Attacks aren't isolated to large cities either, they can also target services in smaller towns. Jeraj (2022) reported that the Redcar and Cleveland Council (Redcar is a small town in North Yorkshire, UK), was hit by a catastrophic attack that took down the entire network and systems in a matter of minutes.

It wasn't just the Council's computers that were affected: phones and other devices connected to the network were rendered unusable. Even visitors to the website were met with error messages. The Council had become another victim of a ransomware attack.

So, what made these attacks possible? These breaches weren't the result of a hacker breaking through some firewall or exploiting a vulnerability in out-of-service software. The attack was the result of an employee clicking on an attachment in a phishing email.

But – you're not the sort of person who'd fall for something as silly as a phishing email, right? This also happens to be what people who clicked on phishing emails thought, before they fell victim.

One of the main reasons why those working in social care are such high value targets for cybercriminals is because very few other people know about the information they hold. It's information that can be used to create extremely convincing attacks.

Common misconceptions

'If we classify the attacks made using social engineering techniques under the titles of "Computer Hacking"' and "Fraud", these incidents form an important portion of crimes' (Mataracioglu & Ozkan, 2012, p. 2). Nevertheless, it can be difficult to convince a person that they are at risk of becoming a victim.

Hadlington (2017) found that, even when a person has been convinced they are still at risk of making mistakes, a positive attitude towards cybersecurity in organisations has still been related to risky cybersecurity behaviours in the past.

As we learn more about the techniques that make cyberattacks so successful, cybercriminals advance their methods. As a result, even someone who is confident in their attitude towards security is still at risk.

Muncaster (2015) reported on research conducted on over 1,000 members of organisations through a self-assessment: 58 per cent of respondents said they were aware of security threats and the risk they pose to corporate information. However, at the same time 39 per cent of the respondents thought that it was the company's responsibility to protect data. And 62 per cent of respondents said they thought their behaviour had a low to moderate impact on the corporation's security. Additionally, 48 per cent claimed they weren't bothered about their corporate security policy, as they did not believe it affected their role.

Muncaster exemplifies one of the most common issues with self-assessment: the belief that we know more than we really do. When it comes to cybersecurity, people often hold misconceptions about the capabilities of cybercriminals and their role in stopping them.

Even people who think they have a good knowledge of cybersecurity can have misconceived notions regarding their place and position towards the safety of the organisation they work for and the data held. For you to become secure and mitigate the risk to your patients and colleagues throughout your career, it is vital to recognise your place in keeping data safe.

However, I urge you not to see such responsibility in a negative light. Instead, see responsibility and pressure as a privilege. You are entrusted with helping to protect valuable information from falling into the wrong hands. To do so you need to empower yourself with a working knowledge of cybersecurity, one you can apply to everyday practices and procedures. So, let's examine what that should look like.

How to be secure

So how do we reduce the risk of falling victim to an attack? 'It is not enough to just publish policies and expect them to read, understand and implement what is required' (Kumar, et al., 2015, p. 18).

You need training, education, and awareness in order to change behaviour by developing and maintaining a secure culture. How these different concepts feed into each other is vital for understanding how to develop your level of security.

Training, education, and awareness

I want to cover exactly what training, education, and awareness mean as they pertain to cybersecurity.

- **Training**: Imparting knowledge of how to do a certain action through practice and reinforcement.
- **Education**: Teaching the knowledge of a subject, which can be built upon in greater detail with further education.
- **Awareness**: Understanding what connects actions to the intended or unintended consequences of those actions – which can be gained through education and training.

Cybersecurity awareness is what we're aiming for, because you need to know how your actions will impact your level of security. From his research into security policies, Alkhurayyif (2019) determined that a person's understanding of security policies will depend upon the readability of the content. You need to begin with education of the subject matter at its most foundational level, then build with training, and continue this process in order to gain the level of awareness you need.

Let's look at a quick hypothetical example.

It is not enough simply to know that phishing emails will try to manipulate you into clicking on a button, or performing a certain action. You need to recognise the techniques that cybercriminals use in phishing emails in order to manipulate you. You need to understand how they will use information they can find out about you online to tailor their attack specifically to you – using people you know and subjects that are of interest to you.

You then need to practise the action of spotting phishing emails to be sure that you will be able to detect them when genuine attacks come into your inbox. This training will help you find out if there are certain areas of the subject that you are struggling with, allowing you to go and educate further in these areas.

Understanding one area of cybersecurity requires a holistic approach to the matter. For example, an awareness of phishing and spear-phishing means you understand what your digital footprint is, and how it impacts your susceptibility to these types of attack. You need to be sure to maintain the level of information you make public about your life. This means your digital footprint doesn't contain information that can be used by a cybercriminal to create a targeted attack against you.

To understand what impact each piece of information you share can have on your digital footprint you need to know about Open Source Intelligence (OSINT): this is often how cybercriminals begin their attacks. They perform reconnaissance on their target by collecting information online. You need to know how your actions online impact how convincing an attack made against you can be.

There are many more of your daily practices that you need to apply this same thinking to – not just when it comes to checking your emails.

Level of understanding

Applying your knowledge means more than simply being able to recite some information you've read in a book. Bloom's *Taxonomy of Educational Objectives* (Bloom, 1969) states that learners should be successful if they have sufficient time and support. In order to reach the desired outcome, each individual's required amount of time and support differs.

In *Revising Bloom's Taxonomy*, Anderson and Krathwohl (2002) argue that learners should be judged against clear objectives rather than competitive systems. This is because categorising learners as successful or unsuccessful based on where their scores lie in comparison with others doing the same course detracts from the objective of understanding the matter at hand.

Vasileiou & Furnell (2019) outlined six levels of understanding, which we will use to conclude the level of understanding you should reach.

1   **Remembering:** *The ability to retrieve, recognise and recall information from the course. A* simple quiz can prove this. Remembering what to do if a data

breach occurs means you know how to handle the situation, as well as how to escalate and report it further.

2   **Understanding:** *The ability to construct meaning from the course and interpret, classify, summarise, compare, or explain teachings.* Can be proven by you being able to show a full table of advantages and disadvantages. Do you appreciate the damage to reputation and impact a breach may have?

3   **Applying:** *The ability to use knowledge in a defined situation or simulation.* This ability can be confirmed by being able to identify the appropriate methods to deal with possible cybersecurity scenarios. Do you take precautions? Do you lock desktops and devices? Do you watch out for 'tailgaters'? Are you incorporating this into your normal daily activities?

4   **Analysing:** *Can break material up into parts and understand how these parts interact with each other to provide an overall purpose.* Can compare and ascertain how specific case studies are similar or dissimilar and why their results were different. Are you able to assess and analyse a situation? Do you click on links in a rush without thinking? Can you identify cybersecurity vulnerabilities in a peer's behaviour?

5   **Evaluating:** *Can make judgements based on the information and standards provided.* You should be able to create a model, table, or method of comparison to understand how to support or disprove concepts and demonstrate findings. Are you able to identify issues that cause cybersecurity vulnerabilities by staff circumnavigating policies and procedures? Do systems need to be revisited to become more secure?

6   **Creating:** *Can put elements together to form a full concept of a topic, including the planning, generating of ideas, and production.* You should be able to provide a detailed plan of how the future of cybersecurity may be. Are you able to create a better cybersecurity culture? Are you able to develop security policies and procedures in future projects?

Naturally, the ideal scenario would be for everyone to reach the highest level of understanding in this taxonomy. However, in reality, this will probably not be reached by all. Nevertheless, it's vital that everyone reaches the level of 'Analysing'.

Let's take video conferencing as an example. One of the biggest misconceptions is that using these services or starting a chat through social media sites is safe enough because the website or application is encrypted. This shows a lack of understanding across several elements of security. For starters, just because a website or app is encrypted doesn't mean it is unhackable or people can't access content being transmitted. In fact, any amount of time looking into many of the most popular video conferencing services will show a plethora of examples of hackers entering into conference calls the users believed were secure.

The service will probably say it is encrypted, but that does not mean data transmitted is protected from end-to-end. As a result, people have transmitted valuable and personal information through services that can easily be accessed by cybercriminals. Did you know that the more people who are on a video conference call the less secure it becomes? Services that do offer complete end-to-end encryption are often unable to extend this beyond 1-to-1 phone calls.

To understand why all of this is such an issue for those working in your industry is to understand how valuable the information you are talking about is. Should someone enter into a conversation without you knowing, and they record what is being discussed, they will have valuable intel that can be used to spearhead sophisticated cyberattacks. As we have seen, the victims who pay the biggest price are often the most vulnerable: the very people who trusted you.

Developing culture by changing behaviour

It is not easy to change people's behaviour. In fact it is one of the most difficult aspects of security training. Yes, someone might perform the correct action within a controlled setting like a training simulation, but that doesn't mean their behaviour is actually going to be any different going forward. They've simply done what they needed to do in order to pass a tick-box exercise so they can move on, without implementing secure behaviours into their daily practices.

Habits are tough to break, and instilling new ones is almost impossible if the person doesn't believe in why they're doing them. It's hard enough to get people to exercise more and eat better even when we know the benefits of these habits are happier and healthier lives. Imagine trying to instil behavioural changes in a person who doesn't even think they apply to them.

This is why cybersecurity awareness is so important. It means a person recognises why they need to change their behaviour, because they understand what the consequences of the right and the wrong actions are.

Let's play out an example we can all relate to.

Once upon a time, seat belts were not in cars. Then one day cars started having them fitted, but they weren't mandatory, and many people didn't use them. One day it was decided that they should be made mandatory, and still there were those who did not put on their seat belt.

Their behaviour was ingrained into them, and to give up their behaviour, concede there was a better way, and then perform this new action consistently took a long time. However, nowadays we would consider it unusual for a person to get into a vehicle and *not* put on their seat belt.

Nowadays putting on our seat belts is simply part of the process of using a vehicle. The behaviour is a habit. This is precisely what secure behaviours need to be within your life, they must become habits that you do as part of the process of work. Rather than unwelcome additions to your responsibilities: secure behaviours need to be an intrinsic element of them.

We can take this example a step further. There are expected actions that we all take when we come to traffic lights in a vehicle or cross the road. One person flouting these rules would create chaos for everybody else. Now while it's quite easy to imagine the chaos that could be caused by a lorry driver flouting these rules, it's harder to imagine when it comes to cybersecurity.

Nevertheless, the consequences of flouting security are not ethereal; they are just as real. As we have seen from the examples already discussed, the impact of practices not being secure can be severe. Worst of all, these consequences so often fall at the feet of those most vulnerable.

What an effective security culture looks like

The European Union Agency for Network and Information Security (ENISA) states that an effective cybersecurity culture:

> encompasses familiar topics including cybersecurity awareness and information security frameworks but is broader in both scope and application, being concerned with making information security considerations an integral part of an employee's job, habits and conduct, embedding them in their day-to-day actions.
>
> (ENISA, 2018, p. 5)

In an article for the journal *Computers and Security*, Da Veiga and Eloff (2010), outline the seven elements of security culture known as the Security Culture Framework. Using these, we can better understand the human factors that contribute to an effective security culture.

1   Behaviours
2   Attitudes
3   Cognitions
4   Compliance
5   Communication
6   Norms
7   Responsibilities

Assessing these different elements of security provides insight into where the weaknesses and the strengths are. From this information an effective plan can be put in place to tackle the issues inhibiting security. While this assessment is used to evaluate an organisation, it also provides a great starting point for you to assess your own beliefs and daily practices.

Don't simply assess these factors at the start of your security journey and stop there. Continue to measure yourself during your training. With the wealth of competing priorities you have, it's vital your time is spent as effectively as possible. It's important to assess your progress and where you can still improve, as this will help you to ensure the time you spend will be spent effectively.

Cybersecurity is constantly advancing, as new methods of deception are devised by cybercriminals, we counter, and so the cycle continues. Your training and assessments are designed to prepare you against the latest threats, and to empower you with knowledge enabling you to choose the right actions. Security is by no means a bad thing, rather than simply a shield to defend yourself, it is a sword for you to protect the vulnerable in your care.

It is important to have a positive view of cybersecurity. Too often security becomes about saying 'No', you can't do this or you shouldn't do that. However, this creates a very warped view of what security is all about. Instead, flip this perspective so the focal point is a positive one. Security is about empowering you with the knowledge and skills to help protect yourself and better maintain the bond of trust that has been given to you by those in your care.

When you operate out of a positive paradigm, cybersecurity becomes a welcome aid, not an unwelcome addition to your role. By an entire organisation operating out of this paradigm, members throughout will buy into incorporating secure behaviours into their daily practices, helping to develop and maintain a security culture.

So you can understand this better, let's play out another example using one of the key elements of cybersecurity, password protection.

Across an organisation people are using personal information that can be found online to create passwords. As we covered previously, information such as social media is part of your digital footprint, which cybercriminals can use to decipher passwords. Now let's say people are also reusing these passwords across multiple accounts, if one account's password is discovered then all the other accounts are at risk too.

These are common examples of behaviours that aren't secure. If such behaviours are being allowed in the workplace it is likely that multiple people will be doing it, fostering a culture of insecurity. This culture will impact the ways in which other actions are performed. Instead of only communicating personal information safely though phone call or in person, people may use social media or messaging apps to send the information between each other.

The longer a culture of insecurity is allowed to grow, the more behaviours will become insecure. As this culture is allowed to foster it becomes more difficult to change people's behaviours in order to create a secure culture.

In a secure culture what would people's passwords look like? First, they wouldn't use personal information to make them memorable. Thanks to their education and training they would be aware of how basing passwords on personal information makes them susceptible to deciphering, because cybercriminals can find the information they need from their digital footprint through OSINT.

Instead, passwords would be created using random words, this means they are secure and memorable. For example, TwoBr!rds1Stone is easy to remember and is not based on personal information.

They would also not reuse passwords across multiple accounts. They would be aware of how this could lead to several accounts being compromised if the password is discovered.

But remember, an effective cybersecurity culture is a positive one. As a result, the messaging would not be framed as you can't use personal information, or you can't reuse passwords. Rather, you can protect those in your care by using genuinely random passwords that cybercriminals can't guess; or you can protect multiple accounts using different passwords for each.

Now when it comes to passwords, there is another layer of security that a secure culture would have instilled within people. People would be using password managers and Multi-Factor Authentication (MFA).

Password managers store passwords, this means they can be incredibly random. They can even come up with passwords so you don't have to. MFA adds an additional layer of security over the account because, if someone were to uncover the password, they still wouldn't be able to enter the account without the second code. MFA is like having two locks on your door, if someone was to get hold of one key, they still wouldn't be able to get through the door without the other.

Key behaviours, like secure password practices, require education and training for an awareness of the consequences of using weak or strong passwords to be developed. Otherwise, a person will not buy into the idea of incorporating these behaviours into their daily practices.

Clearing the first hurdle

When it comes to cybersecurity, what is most important is often the most difficult: convincing people that it actually matters to them. I've tried to use real-world examples of the consequences of bad security practices in order to show the impact negligence towards cybersecurity leads to.

The truth is that, when you work with people's personal information, you are a target. You might not see monetary value in the sensitive information you are responsible for, but that doesn't mean other people can't.

You might not think of yourself as worth attacking because you don't have access to financial records, or have privileged access within a network. However, your account operates within a network that is full of sensitive information. It does not matter whether you have access to a lot or a little, gaining that first step into a network is enough for many cybercriminals to do damage.

By understanding the value of personal information and why you are a target, you will have cleared the first hurdle. Hopefully, this chapter has gone some way towards highlighting how treating the information you are entrusted with in a responsible way is an intrinsic part of the role you have within the lives of those who trust you.

Once you recognise that cybersecurity matters, you need to understand how to strengthen your defences. This means making processes more secure, from how you communicate sensitive information with colleagues to the platforms you use to conduct virtual meetings and sessions. All aspects of your daily practices need to be conducted securely.

There can be no exceptions within security – this is why we include the physical information you record within this same umbrella. Cybercriminals don't care where the information comes from, they care about the fact they can get their hands on it.

Garnering a collective buy-in towards making daily practices more secure is difficult within an organisation. There are those who will resist and those who will be more onboard. By promoting the benefits changes in behaviour will bring, an organisation can begin to develop their culture into a secure one.

However, for any culture to last it needs to be maintained. You cannot accelerate up to 70 mph, take your foot off the accelerator, and expect to maintain your speed. You will slow down, lose momentum, and eventually come to a standstill once again.

In the same way, if the hard work has been done and a security culture has finally been established it only makes sense to maintain it. This means updating training to keep up with the latest trends and types of attacks, making sure training is revisited, and concepts are refreshed. Educate new starters so they are aware of what platforms are safe to use and the secure way to store and communicate information.

Most importantly of all, make sure everyone understands the value in secure behavioural practices and the benefits brought by improving cybersecurity. People need to understand the *why* behind a change. It is not simply for the organisation, but for those who are most vulnerable – so they don't end up paying the price.

References

Aldawood, H., & Skinner, G. (2019). Reviewing cyber security social engineering training and awareness programs: Pitfalls and ongoing issues. *Future Internet, 11*(*3*), 73. https://doi.org/10.3390/fi11030073.

Alkhurayyif, Y. (2019). *Evaluating readability as a factor in information security policies [Doctoral dissertation].* https://stax.strath.ac.uk/concern/parent/vt150j43d/file_sets/05741s05x.

Anderson, L.W., & Krathwohl, D.R. *et al.* (2001). *A Taxonomy for Learning, Teaching, and Assessing: A Revision of Bloom's Taxonomy of Educational Objectives.* Boston, MA: Allyn & Bacon (Pearson Education Group).

Armour, R. (2022, March 22). Top Scottish charity compromised by cyber-attack as data is dumped on dark web. *Third Force News.* https://tfn.scot/news/top-scottish-charity-compromised-by-cyber-attack-as-data-is-dumped-on-dark-web#:~:text=SAMH%20had%20posted%20a%20notice,data%20on%20the%20dark%20web

Barth, S., & De Jong, M.D. (2017). The privacy paradox: Investigating discrepancies between expressed privacy concerns and actual online behavior – A systematic literature review. *Telematics and Informatics, 34*(*7*), 1038–1058. https://doi.org/10.1016/j.tele.2017.04.013.

Bloom, B.S. (1969). *Taxonomy of Educational Objectives: The Classification of Educational Goals.* Boston, MA: Addison-Wesley Longman.

Chaudhry, A., Crowcroft, J., Howard, H., Madhavapeddy, A., Mortier, R., Haddadi, H., & McAuley, D. (2015). Personal data: Thinking inside the box. *Aarhus Series on Human Centered Computing, 1*(*1*). https://doi.org/10.7146/aahcc.v1i1.21312.

Cromer, R., Denneson, L.M., Pisciotta, M., Williams, H., Woods, S., & Dobscha, S.K. (2017). Trust in mental health clinicians among patients who access clinical notes online. *Psychiatric Services, 68*(*5*), 520–523. https://doi.org/10.1176/appi.ps.201600168.

Da Veiga, A., & Eloff, J. (2010). A framework and assessment instrument for information security culture. *Computers & Security, 29*(*2*), 196–207. https://doi.org/10.1016/j.cose.2009.09.002.

ENISA. (2018). *Cyber Security Culture in Organisations.* European Union Agency for Cybersecurity. https://www.enisa.europa.eu/publications/cyber-security-culture-in-organisations/@@download/fullReport.

FINLEX. (2021, December 7). Neglecting the appropriate security of personal data processing and failing to report a data security breach. *Etusivu – FINLEX.* https://finlex.fi/fi/viranomaiset/tsv/2021/20211183. (Reported by WIRED in English.)

Hadlington, L. (2017). Human factors in cybersecurity: Examining the link between internet addiction, impulsivity, attitudes towards cybersecurity, and risky cybersecurity behaviours. *Heliyon*, *3*(7). https://doi.org/10.1016/j.heliyon.2017.e00346.

Halevi, T., Memon, N., & Nov, O. (2015). Spear-phishing in the wild: A real-world study of personality, phishing self-efficacy and vulnerability to spear-phishing attacks. *SSRN Electronic Journal*. https://doi.org/10.2139/ssrn.2544742.

Jeraj, S. (2022, May 3). How ransomware shut down an English council. *New Statesman*. https://www.newstatesman.com/spotlight/cybersecurity/2022/05/how-ransomwa re-shut-down-an-english-council.

Kumar, A., Chaudhary, M., & Kumar, N. (2015). Social engineering threats and awareness: A survey. *European Journal of Advances in Engineering and Technology*, *2*(11), 15–19. https:// citeseerx.ist.psu.edu/document?repid=rep1&type=pdf&doi=2b1b369f8ee40bb1641525314 47b10f59d08cb07.

Mataracioglu, T., & Ozkan, S. (2012). User awareness measurement through social engineering. https://arxiv.org/pdf/1108.2149.pdf.

Muncaster, P. (2022, October 17). Hackney council ransomware attack cost £12m+. *Infosecurity Magazine*. https://www.infosecurity-magazine.com/news/hackney-council-ransom ware-attack/#:~:text=A%20local%20government%20authority%20in,according%20to%20a %20local%20report.

Muncaster, P. (2015, January 13). Cisco: Complacency makes staff major security threat. *Infosecurity Magazine*. https://www.infosecurity-magazine.com/news/complacency-a nd-low-awareness/.

Ralston, W. (2021, May 4). They told their therapists everything. Hackers leaked it all. *WIRED*. https://www.wired.com/story/vastaamo-psychotherapy-patients-hack-data-breach/.

Vasileiou, I., & Furnell, S.M. (2019) *Cybersecurity Education for Awareness and Compliance*. Hershey, PA: IGI Global, 101–120. https://doi.org/10.4018/978-1-5225-7847-5.

6 GDPR and technology

Gary Hibberd and Mike Roberts

Technology and data protection: The requirement for security

The General Data Protection Regulation (2018) (GDPR; https://gdpr-info.eu/) is a regulation put in place by the European Union (EU) to protect the privacy and personal data of EU citizens. It came into effect on 25 May 2018, and it has had a significant impact on the protection of personal data for data subjects, because it speaks directly to organisations of all shapes and sizes about the need for protecting personal data and the responsibility around the use of data.

Companies and organisations that collect, process, and store personal data must comply with the GDPR and the UK Data Protection Act (2018) (DPA; https://www.legislation.gov.uk/ukpga/2018/12/contents/enacted). And there is little doubt that these legal requirements have brought about major changes in the way organisations handle personal data, and technology has played a key role in helping organisations comply with them.

As the UK DPA largely mirrors what is in the EU GDPR, we will set our focus and references on the GDPR, as this has the widest reach, across Europe and EU citizens. But please note that, apart from the specific references, what follows in terms of requirements relates to both the GDPR and the UK DPA.

This is important to note, as there are several parts of the GDPR that are relevant for our discussion, but perhaps the most instructive is Article 32(1), 'Security of Processing', which states:

> Taking into account the state of the art, the costs of implementation and the nature, scope, context and purposes of processing as well as the risk of varying likelihood and severity for the rights and freedoms of natural persons, the controller and the processor shall implement appropriate technical and organisational measures to ensure a level of security appropriate to the risk.
>
> (Article 32)

There are several parts to this worthy of discussion.

From the outset, it states that we must take into account three things when considering the type of security we are implementing when processing data:

DOI: 10.4324/9781003364184-7

- The state of the art.
- The costs of implementation.
- The nature, scope, and context.

Perhaps the most confusing but more relevant of these requirements is the phrase 'the state of the art'. I believe this is where the genius of the GDPR lies, where it is future-proofing itself for the technological changes that are to come. Although the installation and use of technical tools are useful (e.g. antivirus software to prevent infection from computer viruses), it is not saying you must install them, because although they are mechanisms for securing data today, tomorrow there may be another technology. Perhaps biometrics, or artificial intelligence (AI) will become ubiquitous across all devices and technologies. Therefore, what is being asked is that you take into account what is currently at the forefront of capability, and what is the 'state of the art' technology that exists today.

At this point it's important not to panic and think we need to implement costly security, just because it exists. The next two points stated again reveal the adaptability of the GDPR, as they ask us to take into account the costs of implementation based on the nature, scope, and context of the processing. Therefore, every person adhering to the GDPR should ask '*What would be reasonable for me to implement, given the nature of the data I am processing?*'

In addition to these considerations, Article 5 (GDPR) makes a very clear point that it is not just technical controls that should be considered, but organisational measures too, stating that '*the processor shall implement appropriate technical and organisational measures*'.

This word, 'appropriate' appears 116 times in the GDPR, and can be thought to mean suitable or compatible for the situation or person. Therefore, what is appropriate to you, will be different to that it appropriate for an organisation that operates internationally, employees hundreds of technical people, and has offices in a dozen different countries.

This chapter will focus on the technical aspects of the GDPR and what kind of technologies would be considered 'appropriate'. But do not lose sight of the fact that technical controls without organisational controls is simply a recipe for disaster. As the cybersecurity expert and author, Bruce Schneier (2006) said: 'If you think technology can solve your security problems, then you don't understand the problems and you don't understand the technology.'

Thinking we can improve data protection and security with technology alone is like thinking we can improve road safety by making better cars. Everyone understands that a car is neither good nor bad. They can be expensive or cheap. It is the use and maintenance of this 'technology' that dictates whether or not they can do us harm or not.

Only by following the rules of the road can we be sure that our journey is going to be successful, and that our passengers are kept safe. Because, be under no illusion, the landscape is becoming increasingly dangerous with the cost of cybercrime set to continue to rise exponentially over the coming years (Statista, n.d.).

Unless we become safer 'drivers', the likelihood of us becoming victims of cybercrime or causing our own data breach is only ever going to increase.

Appropriate tools

So, what would be deemed to be appropriate in the context of 'technical measures and data protection'? Of course, there are many technical devices and systems we could discuss, but we will focus our attention on the four key areas that I believe are most relevant and of pressing need and interest to this community. These are:

- Encryption
- Email protection
- External devices
- Access control

For the avoidance of doubt, these topics could each fill a volume of their own, and each of them feature at great length in international security standards, such as the International Organization for Standardization (ISO) standard, ISO27001:2022 ((ISO 2022). ISO standards set a benchmark for organisations to implement appropriate security management systems and controls. In these standards, these topics are discussed alongside many others, but my aim is to highlight what I believe are the essential aspects of technical security you need to be aware of, and therefore our attention for the remainder of this book will focus on these topics.

Encryption

Encryption is a way to protect information by converting it into a code that can only be deciphered or read by someone with a special key or password. It is like locking a physical document in a safe, but instead of using a physical lock, encryption uses mathematical algorithms to secure the information. This makes it much harder for someone who is not authorised to access the information to read it.

For example, imagine you have a secret message written on a piece of paper and you want to send it to a friend, but you don't want anyone else to read it. You could use encryption to convert the message into a code that only your friend can read. In order to do so, you would first have to provide your friend with the 'key', in order to decrypt it. Once the message has been received and decrypted, it will be readable to your friend, but to anyone else, it would be just a bunch of letters and numbers that did not make any sense.

Encryption is commonly used to protect sensitive information such as personal data, financial information, and confidential business information. It is used in many aspects of our daily life, from online shopping, banking, and mobile communication to cloud storage, and it's an important tool for companies and organisations to secure their data and comply with regulations such as the GDPR.

Under the GDPR, organisations are required to protect personal data from unauthorised access, alteration, or destruction, and encryption is one of the most effective ways to do this. This is because it makes the data unreadable to anyone who does not hold the appropriate decryption key. Therefore, with the help of encryption, you can secure personal data even if it is lost or stolen. For example:

> Stevie took their car to the garage one late winter evening to fill up on petrol. It had been a long day at the school, talking to many children and parents. Filling up the car, they walked into the station and decided to grab a cup of coffee before paying. As they stood, waiting for the coffee to finish pouring, they looked out to the car they had just left, to see a man opening the rear door, and grabbing their bag, and run off into the darkness. In their exhausted state, they had forgotten to lock the car. The good news? The laptop was encrypted, so no data was lost and therefore the risk had been mitigated and managed effectively.

In fact, there are two types of encryption you should be aware of:

- Encryption at rest
- Encryption in transit

In the example mentioned above, the device that Stevie used allowed the data to be encrypted 'at rest', meaning it is encrypted when on the device. If you are using an Apple mobile device, this enables encryption at rest. Only someone who has access to the passcode on your device can access the information, and anyone who does not, cannot gain access to it.

In fact, the ability to access encrypted information on devices has been a matter of much debate for many years, with Apple and the Federal Bureau of Investigation (FBI) having ongoing battles about the ability to access the encrypted information on devices (see Ethics Unwrapped, n.d.).

Encryption in transit, however, refers to the process of encrypting data as it is transmitted across networks, such as the Internet. This helps to protect the data from being intercepted or accessed by unauthorised parties during transmission.

There are several different methods of encryption in transit, but one of the most commonly used is transport layer security (TLS) and its predecessor, secure sockets layer (SSL). These protocols use a process called 'handshaking' to establish a secure connection between the sender and receiver. During the handshaking process, the sender and receiver agree on a set of encryption protocols and keys to use for the session. Once the session is established, all data sent between the sender and receiver is encrypted using the agreed upon protocols and keys. Of course, all of this happens automatically in the background so you don't have to get involved. If you're wondering when this kind of encryption takes place, take a look at your web browser when using an established website. You'll see that most websites have a small padlock in the address bar, and the acronym 'HTTPS', which means hyper text transfer protocol secure. HTTPS is the secure version of the standard HTTP protocol used on the web. In other words, HTTPS uses TLS to encrypt data sent between a web server and a browser, ensuring that sensitive information, such as login credentials and credit card numbers, are protected from eavesdropping and tampering.

This is why cybersecurity professionals advocate the use of another form of encryption in transit technique, called a VPN (virtual private network), which creates a secure and encrypted connection between the user and the network. This prevents the ability for any unauthorised individuals (e.g. colleagues, cleaners, or criminals) to intercept the transmission, a technique known as a 'man-in-the-middle attack'.

> Stevie sat in the coffee shop, after ordering their usual caramel macchiato with a cookie. Knowing that there was work to be done, they logged onto the free Wi-Fi and began going through their inbox, and the emails that had built up over the past few days. In almost 30 emails, Stevie came across the one from the retail store they used for designer jackets. There were some interesting designs, but would the bank balance allow it? 'Before I go shopping, best check the bank balance.' So that's what they did.
>
> Quickly logging into the bank, they soon established that there was more than enough money in the savings to warrant this little 'impulse' buy. Fifteen minutes later, bank details provided, along with delivery details, the purchase was done. Stevie sat back and smiled as they took a bite of the cookie.
>
> Stevie didn't even notice the young man in the corner of the coffee shop, quietly sipping his coffee as he worked on his PC. He sat back and smiled as he also took a bite of a 'millionaire shortcake', as he watched the information from Stevie's computer pass through his, and then on to its final destination of the bank and the retail store. It had taken him just five minutes to set up his device as a router in the coffee shop. Just to be sure that people would login, he called his device '1-Free-Coffee-WiFi', and made sure anyone connecting would not need to ask for a password. Then he waited until those in the coffee shop started to connect to his device.
>
> Of course, there were those who had a VPN, so the young man in the corner couldn't see what they were transmitting. But when someone didn't use a VPN, he was able to see everything they did on any website they visited. Harvesting names, addresses, passwords, bank account numbers, sort codes, credit card numbers, CVV numbers, expiry dates, and much, much more.

Taking another sip of coffee, the young man in the corner wondered what he would order first, using 'Stevie1974' credit card number?

By using encryption, organisations can show that they have taken appropriate steps to protect personal data, which can be important in the event of an audit or investigation by law enforcement agencies or the Information Commissioners Office (ICO). Encryption should therefore be considered a vital aspect of your security defences. It is also worth noting that encryption is specifically mentioned in the GDPR in several places. When thinking about the software packages and devices you use, you should always consider when, how, and what forms of encryption is used.

The question one should always ask is: 'How can I ensure this information is secured from unauthorised access?'. This question should then be followed by more detailed questions, such as:

- Is the data encrypted at rest?
- How is the data encrypted in transit?
- What forms of encryption are being used?

Dependent on the tool or software you're using, these questions will be more important or less important, so their relevance should still be considered. Of course, you may not always be confident technically to understand the answers to the above, but simply asking will put you in a stronger position and demonstrates that you are taking due care and attention, when purchasing software tools, or devices.

Remember, encryption is a very technical topic, and one that dominates an entire sector of the technology and security sector. But this is for good reason. It is vital in the fight against data breaches and cybercrime.

Email protection

One software tool that utilises encryption is electronic mail, or email as we often refer to it.

Email management is an important aspect of data protection under the GDPR for several reasons, not all of which are linked to the ability to transmit data securely, a topic we shall return to shortly.

Accuracy

Article 5(d) of the GDPR states that personal data shall be

> accurate and, where necessary, kept up to date; every reasonable step must be taken to ensure that personal data that are inaccurate, having regard to the purposes for which they are processed, are erased or rectified without delay ('accuracy').
>
> (GDPR, Article 5(d))

Therefore, the GDPR expects you to ensure that personal data is accurate and up-to-date. Email management can help you to achieve this by automating the process of updating contact details and removing inactive email addresses. This can help to ensure that the personal data being used by you is accurate and up-to-date.

Minimisation and storage limitation

Another important aspect of email management under the GDPR is that it can help organisations to comply with the requirement for 'data minimisation'. The GDPR requires organisations to minimise the amount of personal data they collect and process, and states that personal data shall be: 'adequate, relevant and limited to what is necessary in relation to the purposes for which they are processed' (data minimisation) (GDPR, Article 5c).

Email management can help you to achieve this by automating the process of unsubscribing individuals from mailing lists, which can help to reduce the amount of personal data being held by you. You should also note that the principle requires data to be 'relevant and limited to what is necessary', and therefore care should be taken when considering the information obtained and shared via email.

Why is it important to state this here? Because the use of email has now become so ubiquitous, that we are forgetting that email is a formal form of communication. One that has incredible power and reach, and therefore should be carefully considered and used.

Email is no longer a method of transferring data around the world. It is a data store, and it should be considered as such. Every time you send an email containing personal data, or an attachment with notes, that email sits within your 'Sent' folder, until such time that you decide to erase it. Of course, there are system policies and rules you can define that will automatically archive this information, but this is down to you to determine and set. This is important because another requirement of the GDPR is called 'storage limitation', where it states that personal data shall be:

> Kept in a form which permits identification of data subjects for no longer than is necessary for the purposes for which the personal data are processed; personal data may be stored for longer periods insofar as the personal data will be processed solely for archiving purposes in the public interest, scientific or historical research purposes or statistical purposes in accordance with Article 89 (1) subject to the implementation of the appropriate technical and organisational measures required by this Regulation in order to safeguard the rights and freedoms of the data subject (storage limitation)'
>
> (GDPR, Article5(d))

Note that the principle talks about keeping data for 'no longer than is necessary'. The word necessary is often debated in practices, where people want to know how the ICO has defined this. The simple answer is: they haven't. This is for you to determine and be able to answer the question. Of course, this topic is far wider than this chapter and certainly relates to more than email. But the purpose of discussing it here is to remind you that email must also only be kept for as long as is necessary. Stating that you delete client files after seven years is only going to be accurate if you ensure that any notes or conversations that you had via email are also removed or archived appropriately.

Email encryption

It is at this point that we must again return to the topic of encryption, as the term encryption in transit clearly is something that refers to email. Essentially, email encryption is the method used to protect the content of an email from being intercepted or read by anyone other than the intended recipient. When an email is encrypted, it is converted into a coded message that can only be read by someone with the right 'key' to decrypt it.

There are two main types of email encryption: transport layer security (TLS, mentioned above) and secure/multipurpose Internet mail extensions (S/MIME).

TLS has been discussed above, in relation to the 'handshake' between your device and the website that you use. But it is also the protocol that encrypts email as it travels between the sender's and recipient's email servers, ensuring that any third parties intercepting the email cannot read its contents – which helps to prevent man-in-the-middle attacks.

S/MIME is a security standard for email that allows users to encrypt the message, and also digitally sign their email messages. S/MIME uses public key infrastructure (PKI) technology to encrypt and sign the emails. Each user has a digital certificate that contains their public key, which is used to encrypt the email. The private key, which is known only to the user, is used to decrypt the email.

Both methods ensure that the email is only readable by the intended recipient, but S/MIME provides additional features such as a digital signature, which verifies that the email is truly sent by the person who claims to have sent it. This is becoming increasingly important as the use of phishing emails is on the rise. See, for example, the article 'Email cyberattacks ncreased 48% in first of of 2022' (Security, 2022), where the scammers impersonated someone or an organisation that you know. However, with S/MIME and other forms of digital signatures, you can be confident that the email has come from the trusted individual, and not from scammers or fraudsters.

Some email systems, like Gmail, also offer a technology called 'end-to-end encryption' (E2EE), which encrypts the email on the sender device and decrypts it on the recipient device. This means that any intermediaries (such as email servers or cloud storage providers) that handle the data along the way can only see the encrypted version of the data and cannot read the plain text.

E2EE typically uses a pair of keys, one private and one public, to encrypt and decrypt the data. The private key is kept on the sender's device and is used to encrypt the data and the public key is shared with the intended recipient and used to decrypt the data.

Here is a basic overview of the process:

- The sender's system generates a pair of encryption keys (public and private).
- The sender encrypts the message using the recipient's public key.
- The encrypted message is sent to the recipient.
- The recipient receives the message and decrypts it using their private key.

Popular examples of E2EE are the systems 'Signal' and Proton Mail.

Finally, if no specialist software or rules are applied, then you can also configure your email systems to use 'Opportunistic TLS' which tries to encrypt the email using the strongest method supported by the recipient's email service, thus providing an additional layer of security.

In conclusion, email management is an important aspect of data protection under the GDPR. It can help you to ensure that personal data is accurate, up-to-date, and complies with the Regulation's requirement for data minimisation and storage limitation.

External devices

Almost all of us will use an external device that stores data in one form or another. An external device can include mobile phones, tablets, laptops, external hard drives, or USB drives. The management of external devices therefore is of critical importance to you and to compliance of the GDPR. Also not fully discussed here, it is worth noting that international standards such as ISO27001 (ISO) and many cybersecurity professionals talk about external devices and removable media almost as if they are the same thing, and in some cases there is an overlap.

The risk associated with external devices and removable media is associated to the very reason they exist: they are transportable and therefore their use is very flexible. However, this also means that they are prone to being lost or stolen, and if adequate security has not been applied to them, the data is therefore compromised.

Stories of lost laptops, USB drives, and mobile phones and tablets are almost too numerous to mention, and if the devices are not adequately protected from unauthorised use, the likelihood of a data breach increases exponentially.

Once again, protecting these devices can often come down to the question, 'Was the data encrypted?'. On some of these devices, the data is encrypted at rest as standard. On others, it would need to be enabled and configured to ensure the protection is in place. This is also true of USB drives, which are often used to transfer data to data subjects who have requested copies of their information. This again helps to demonstrate compliance with the requirements of the GDPR.

Finally, external drives are also often used for backing up data, which is a great idea. This ensures that should your primary system become unavailable, you have the means to access client information and data. Again, I would urge you to ensure this information is encrypted, to prevent its loss or theft becoming a further challenge that you would need to overcome.

Access control

One of the fundamental requirements of information security is integrity, meaning trust. Can you trust the person accessing the data? And can the data that you see on screen be trusted? Has it been altered in any way?

In order to obtain, or maintain that trust, you need to ensure that the only systems, services, and people who have access to devices or information are known to you, have been validated, and can be trusted.

One of the ways that cyberattackers take over systems, is by gaining access to lower level systems and then looking for ways to 'elevate' their credentials and therefore their capability. One of the primary causes for data breaches or cyber-incidents caused by people is founded in the fact that they had permissions to access information that they shouldn't (e.g. an admin person having access to your payroll system, when they have no reason to access it).

In many cases, access control can be managed very simply, by using appropriate user names and passwords. But there are occasions where allowing access could leave you in breach of the GDPR and other legislations.

Remote desk support (RDS)

One of the services that you may use is to have your IT systems supported by a third-party company. Perhaps you have a friendly neighbour or family member who is good with technology. If it is the former, then the likelihood is that they will use some form of remote desktop management software, where an administrator can access and control your computer remotely.

But RDS can be bad for data protection because it can increase the risk of unauthorised access to personal data. Remote desktop management can open up an additional attack vector for hackers or other malicious actors. Remote access protocols, such as remote desktop protocol (RDP), may have vulnerabilities that can be exploited by attackers to gain unauthorised access to your computer and the personal data stored on it.

Remote desktop management allows an administrator to access and control a user's computer, including the ability to delete files or make changes to the system. This increases the risk of unintended data loss, especially if the administrator is not properly trained or does not have the appropriate level of access to personal data.

But even if there isn't a malicious actor out there looking to do you ill, it's important to note that should you hand over access to your device to a third party, then they have the same level of access to the device as you do. This means that any and all case notes that you have will be accessible by the support person. Simply asking them 'not to look' will not work and is possibly more dangerous, as we know human curiosity will take over.

In short, remote desktop management can be bad for data protection because it increases the risk of unauthorised access, lack of control over who has access to personal data, difficulties in complying with regulations, and data loss. This needs to be considered carefully before making any decisions on who will support you and how you will control access to the data your process.

Conclusion

I have already highlighted the point that, under GDPR Article 32, Security of Processing, there is a need for organisational and technical security measures, but it is important also to state that the GDPR identifies three key aspects of information security that it expects organisations like yours to implement. These are known as the information security triad (or CIA):

Confidentiality
Integrity
Availability

GDPR Article 32(b) states that organisations should have 'the ability to ensure the ongoing confidentiality, integrity, availability and resilience of processing systems and services'.

There are many different aspects of the GDPR that impact information security. For example, the use of data anonymisation. Anonymisation is the process of removing personal identifiers from data so that they can no longer be used to identify an individual. Under the GDPR, you are required to minimise the amount of personal data collected and processed, and anonymisation is just one of many ways to achieve this. For example, using anonymisation you can continue to use data for research and analysis without compromising individual privacy.

Technology and the use of software can also play a key role in helping you comply with the GDPR's requirement for data access and transparency. Under the GDPR, individuals have the right to access their personal data and to know how it is being used. You are required to provide this information in a timely manner and in a format that is easy to understand. By using specific pieces of software you can automate the process of responding to data access requests and removing third-party information, making it easier to comply with the Regulation and requests.

Technology and software can also help you comply with the GDPR's requirement for data breaches. For example, under the GDPR, you are required to report data breaches to the relevant authorities within 72 hours of becoming aware of them, as described in GDPR Article 82. Organisations can detect data breaches quickly and respond to them appropriately if and where technological interventions are added or used, which can also help with notifying affected individuals and the relevant authorities.

Technology in its many forms, including software and applications, plays a key role in helping organisations comply with the GDPR. It can enable organisations to encrypt and anonymise personal data, automate data access and transparency requests, detect data breaches, and adopt privacy-by-design principles. As technology itself, including the software programs it can run, continues to evolve, it is likely that it will play an even greater role in protecting personal data and helping organisations comply with the GDPR.

You are responsible for protecting data (in all its forms) on behalf of the people you are helping or providing a service to. This responsibility cannot be outsourced or passed to someone else, however, you can gain some assistance with the use of applications or programs. This is why the seventh principle of Article 5 is of critical importance, as it states: 'The controller shall be responsible for, and be able to demonstrate compliance with, paragraph 1 (accountability).'

The six principles of the GDPR, and this last statement that I call the seventh principle, are non-negotiable in terms of application to your business. The above statement is a clear statement that not only are you, the controller, responsible for the compliance, but you must also be able to demonstrate it. This chapter should hopefully shine some light on the 'how' to process in your line of work.

Supplementary section on Email

Email security: An introduction

This supplementary section by Mike Roberts of Frama (UK) Ltd takes a closer look at email – one of the most popular methods of digital communication. Its prevalence and security vulnerabilities also make it appealing for cyberattacks such as phishing, domain spoofing, and business email compromise (BEC).

Email

Until it happens to you or someone you know, most people pay little attention to the risks of conducting important business or personal transactions using simple email, only to have its content or delivery challenged after the fact.

The more you dig deeper into the world of email, the more horror stories you hear about the damages caused by email content alterations and disputes arising over delivery, snooping, and fraudulent activities. It's a scary world out there, but this chapter has not been written to worry you, it's to inform you about how to stay safe.

Encryption

Here's my explanation of an email being sent in *very* simple terms.

You send your email, and it travels across the World Wide Web like a postcard written in pencil. The information is most likely more than accessible to scammers, hackers, and cybercriminals waiting to cherry-pick the data for fraudulent purposes.

An email was never designed to be secure and, to this day, the technology remains very much the same. Applying 'end-to-end' encryption to your emails means that the information is secure all the way through that digital journey. I started my journey into the world of email security back in 2016, after discovering a simple, automated encrypted email delivery system called Frama RMail. Within months, I became the digital marketing and sales specialist for this amazing software at Frama (UK) Limited.

Securing your emails sounds simple right? But when most people start exploring the world of encryption keys, public key infrastructure digital certificates and crypto-wrapping widgets, it can be massively off-putting. As can these words no doubt!

The constant challenge for IT professionals and security experts is to balance security and useability. If the most secure system is too complicated or cumbersome to use, people will circumvent it.

IT professionals often underestimate just how simple the user experience must be for widespread adoption. Receiving a link in an email forcing the recipient to set up an account to access an email is not simple enough. Nor is exchanging digital certificates and saving them to a device.

When the recipient says to the sender, 'Just send the darn thing', because they get frustrated with the more secure process, the sender often just sends it, frustrated that they are frustrating the recipient with some policy or process IT has put in place.

If it is not simple to use, people will circumvent the process; and they do – even those who know they shouldn't.

But in today's modern world, solutions are now available that give you the security you need, while also making it simple and easy to use.

So how do we make email secure, and what else do we need to consider?

The words that spring to mind to me are 'forensically provable'. This might not mean much to most but, in its simplest form, this means that I want my sensitive emails to be secure, but I also want *proof* of what was inside that email, when it was sent, proof it was secure, and proof it was delivered and opened.

To me, this covers me for everything. Printing off emails from your sent folder doesn't prove anything. These can be edited, rewritten, date changed, and more – so being able to be forensically secure means everything.

This all comes down to having what's known as a registered receipt. It's what I receive when sending an email using the Frama RMail Outlook plugin. A simple red button that sits inside my Outlook workspace (it also works with Gmail), allows me to create an email, compose the contents, add attachments, and send, but this red button delivers my email through a secure 'pathway', while also ensuring that the delivery status and contents are tracked.

My registered email is then sent to me several hours later with all of the court-admissible proof I need. Simple, yet very powerful.

Because let's face it, in today's modern world, we need simplicity. There's far too much digital pollution out there, and the simpler we make it for ourselves and our recipients, the better.

Have you ever received an email that was encrypted, and then been asked to 'sign up for an account', log in, retrieve the information, download, or, even worse, attach various software solutions to your desktop – all just to receive an email? It's not a pleasant experience.

If you want me to go into technical details, and if you're interested in TLS, PKI, Pretty Good Privacy (PGP), and all the various forms of encryption out there, then feel free to get in touch with me. I'll happily explain this, but what it really comes down to, is that the people I speak to need something that they can use easily, without changing anything in terms of the recipient's experience.

Before I end this chapter, let me give you a typical example of what I hear in my job. I often speak to a therapist who has never used email encryption before. Why would they? They've never had a 'data breach' occur, and therefore, surely it can't happen to them. And then one day, all of a sudden, some sensitive data about their client has been exposed. And it all originated from an email (either being sent to the wrong person or snooped upon by a hacker, who then uses this for blackmail purposes/fraudulent activities). Now this therapist needs email encryption. Great, they are now securing their emails, but this is a *reactive* process on their part, rather than *proactive*. The damage is done, in terms of ICO fines and their reputation.

However, people are turning to secure email more commonly these days, which is a great thing, and I would highly recommend those of you reading this to do the same.

References

Data Protection Act Legislation (UK) (2018) https://www.legislation.gov.uk/ukpga/2018/12/contents/enacted.

Ethics Unwrapped. (n.d.) FBI & Apple Security vs. Privacy. McCombs School of Business: https://ethicsunwrapped.utexas.edu/case-study/fbi-apple-security-vs-privacy.

GDPR (2018). https://gdpr-info.eu/.

GDPR, Article 5. https://gdpr-info.eu/art-5-gdpr/.

GDPR, Article 5c, Data Minimisation. https://gdpr-info.eu/art-5-gdpr.

GDPR, Article 5(d), Storage Limitation. https://gdpr-info.eu/art-5-gdpr.

ICO. https://ico.org.uk/.

ICO, Guide to Data Protection. https://ico.org.uk/for-organisations/guide-to-data-protection/guide-to-the-general-data-protection-regulation-gdpr/security.

ISO (2022). ISO27001:2022. https://www.iso.org/standard/82875.html.

Proton Mail. https://proton.me/.

Schneir, B. (2006, 17 October). The Limits of Technology. https://www.schneier.com/books/a-hackers-mind/.

in a blog post on his website on October 17, 2006, "The Limits of Technology" Security (2022). https://www.securitymagazine.com/articles/98145-email-cyberattacks-increased-48-in-first-half-of-2022.

Statista (n.d.). Chart: Cybercrime Expected to Skyrocket in Coming Years. https://www.statista.com/chart/28878/expected-cost-of-cybercrime-until-2027/.

Weblinks for ICO articles cited in text

Article 5. https://ico.org.uk/media/about-the-ico/disclosure-log/2014536/irq0680151-disclosure.pdf.

Article 32, Security of Processing. https://ico.org.uk/media/about-the-ico/disclosure-log/2014536/irq0680151-disclosure.pdf.

Article 32, p. 64. https://ico.org.uk/media/about-the-ico/disclosure-log/2014536/irq0680151-disclosure.pdf.

Article 82. https://ico.org.uk/media/about-the-ico/disclosure-log/2014536/irq0680151-disclosure.pdf.

7 Safe and secure spaces in digital therapy delivery

Kim Page

Introduction

Online therapy is the way of the future.

'Online therapy is rapidly becoming more available due to improvements in technology, user experience, and slowly reduced internal barriers' (Weinberg et al., 2022, p. 36). Its convenience and accessibility are unmatched. But as we move more and more of our lives into the digital space, we leave a trail of personal data that may be less private than we'd expect. The advancement of information technology (IT) and our reliance on it for everyday life are growing exponentially faster than our regulatory bodies can manage to keep up with.

Few of us realise the extent to which our personal information is available on the Internet, even though breaches of this data happen daily. So, what happens when our online presence ventures beyond the social, beyond the financial, and into the therapeutic? Losing the privacy of a credit card number is one thing – losing the privacy of our deepest thoughts, fears, and inner workings is another entirely.

As a therapist, you already centralise the importance of confidentiality. You've sworn to uphold the code of ethics and defend your clients' privacy to maintain the integrity of the therapeutic relationship and the integrity of the profession as a whole. You keep documents behind several locks. You keep client concerns strictly between you and your supervisor. You soundproof your office to keep voices in and distractions out. But virtual therapy requires its own set of ethics, practices, and protections in order for confidentiality to be upheld. While a universally applied framework for the use of technology is not yet available, we have the experience and the technological standards to rely on, that might create such a framework (see, for example, Kate Anthony, and D. Merz Nagel *Therapy Online: A Practical Guide*, 2010). If you're using technology to communicate with clients, deliver therapy sessions, or maintain records, understanding cybersecurity and best practice is essential. Essential because technology is a core component in every interaction now, and its use is pressing upon the trust and ethics that are foundational. Our opportunity is to develop services on the basis of adopted best practice, not retrospective change driven from risk and error.

DOI: 10.4324/9781003364184-8

The burden you carry

As a therapist in private practice, you're more than just a therapist. You're a business manager, marketer, scheduling manager, client advocate, record-keeper, and you may even be your own accountant. You are also a guardian, a data controller/gatekeeper – and your patient is relying on you. Now that clients are seeking services online, you're scrambling to learn SEO (search engine optimisation), build your website, and rank higher on Google. Amidst all the goings-on of running a business, it can sometimes feel like you don't even have the time to do what you were trained and certified to do: practise therapy.

It is likely you will also be thinking about the lifestyle you'll be able to sustain, including the financial implications for you and any family members and planning for retirement. You'll be considering your skills carefully and will need to think about how well they transfer to an online setting (Worley-James, 2022). And, in addition, you cannot fail to be concerned about the rate of change in technology and how you are accountable for the services you provide, especially the impact this has on the people you work with.

> Needless to say, a global health crisis, worldwide political unrest, and a monumental increase in demand for therapy are enough to magnify a private practitioner's stress. Adding to that stress, the shift away from in-person therapy towards digital means, 'there is now an ephemeral space with no physical limits and many unknown technological factors, such as where on a hard drive material actually goes when it is stored, to contend with'.
>
> (Anthony & Nagel, 2022, p. 58)

So, who has the time for keeping up with the 'wild west' that is cyberspace? In running your business, caring for your clients, and maintaining your mental health, your cup may feel like it's running dry. The financial burden of paying for things like practice management software and compliance fees hasn't made cybersecurity a particularly attractive duty either. These are decisions you were hardly trained to make.

This chapter implores you to adequately educate yourself as a provider of online therapy services. Having an IT professional on your team of staff is not enough in itself. Even though regulations lag behind the pace of technology's capabilities, there's still plenty you can do to keep a client's information safe, give them the privacy they deserve – and protect your own livelihood.

It is time to refocus the conversation over and above the requirements of the General Data Protection Regulation (2018) (GDPR), and give due care to the consideration that technology in a therapy setting needs to be subject to a quality standard. You will find that you will need to assess and adapt as technology changes – to protect your business, your registration, and your past and future clients. Even current efforts to understand burnout are understood to be affected by difficulties with online confidentiality and navigation of telehealth practices and ethical practices (Litam, Ausloos, & Harrichand, 2021).

How we got here

The Internet became widely accessible and popular in the mid-1990s when the development of audio, visual, and data technologies connected individuals from everywhere in the world. Since then, we've seen the rise of video therapy, mental health apps, and therapy during the time of COVID-19. But even before the mental health tech boom of the 2010s and 2020s, therapists had been conducting therapy in remote or asynchronous formats (Situmorang, 2020). Known as 'distance counselling', these therapy sessions began with phone calls or video calls.

When the Internet came onto the scene, therapists had the opportunity to provide additional distance services including instant messaging, live chats, text messaging, video conferencing, and email. Therapists used video platforms like Skype for virtual sessions until 1996, when the United States passed the Health Insurance Portability and Accountability Act (HIPAA), (Rauch, 2018). Since then, therapists have sought more secure video platforms, and apps such as Talkspace and Better Help emerged to connect clients with clinicians for online virtual therapy sessions.

In early 2020, the COVID-19 pandemic became a traumatic event for individuals around the world. While in lockdown, virtual therapy was no longer just *an* option – it was the *only* option. The market for online therapy exploded, not only for mental health apps but also for private practitioners with virtual therapy capabilities.

Therapists saw an influx of clients struggling with health anxiety, grief, unemployment, and economic recession; clients who they had to provide care for while also striving to cultivate their own resilience in the face of potential burnout. So much so, this has become an important area to be understood (BACP, 2021).

Amid a dire need for mental healthcare, clinicians reported also seeing an increase in clients presenting with eating disorders, addictions, substance abuse and misuse, racial trauma, and general stress and being overwhelmed. They also noted an increase in the diversity of client demographics, claiming to see more young people and men who were now open to seeking therapy as a result of the growing de-stigmatisation of a need for therapy.

These circumstances created a perfect storm for overwhelming demand. Of therapists who were surveyed, 80 per cent reported a demand for treatment that caused long waiting lists and overflow referrals. Therapy, and especially online therapy, was bigger than ever before.

Advantages of virtual therapy

At the time of the COVID-19 pandemic, video sessions extended a lifeline to individuals whose care otherwise would have been halted due to pandemic-related restrictions. In a nation with 'one of the highest Internet penetration rates in the world' (Statista, 2022), online therapy was an easy and viable alternative to in-person sessions. For individuals who were already engaged in therapy, the shift to video was a necessary step for continuity of care. For those who had never been in therapy, the video format offered a new, attractive modality to receive comfort and support during a tough time. In the new norm of social isolation, people sought human connection more than ever – and they were willing to experiment with new avenues to obtain it.

Studies conducted prior to the pandemic have already indicated that online counselling may be a superior option for individuals struggling with social isolation. According to analyses documented in 2000 and 2006, clients 'who experienced uneasiness and social separation were more likely to create deep connections through online/cyber counselling than through in-person counselling' (Situmorang, 2020). In a mass isolating event, such as the COVID-19 pandemic, one could argue that online therapy served as more than just a temporary alternative to make do with – it was the most effective form of treatment.

When it comes to treating depression and anxiety, studies have also shown that online cognitive behaviour therapy proves to be just as effective as in-person therapy (Weinberg et al., 2022). For those who may have been hesitant to begin therapy out of resistance to emotional intimacy, online therapy is again a viable solution. Situmorang (2020) notes, 'Clients taking part in online/cyber counselling are less likely to feel powerless for revealing their individual data and also feel less ashamed about their issues, due to the anonymity related to online/cyber counselling.' For those suffering from social phobias (whether pandemic-induced or not), online therapy opens a door to starting treatment and receiving a diagnosis earlier. In a world without remote therapy options, a client's symptoms may create a barrier to ever pursuing treatment in the first place.

Virtual therapy's most notable advantages are in its accessibility, not only for clients presenting with social interaction and outside phobias (for example, agoraphobia) but also for clients whose in-person therapy attendance is limited or made challenging by, for example, an issue of physical mobility. People with disabilities and those without accessible vehicles may have difficulty getting to facility-based healthcare appointments. Especially in the time of COVID-19, an individual relying on a carer for transportation may have additional limitations in their availability for rides to appointments because of social distancing requirements.

Attendance becomes even more challenging if an individual lives far away from the nearest therapy provider and geography can be yet another challenge when a specific skill set in short supply is needed. In this way, online therapy expands access to clients who live in rural or under-served areas (Young & Edwards, 2020). In addition, increasing access to a wider range of demographic groups helps with the destigmatisation of therapy among these groups. All positive, if sometimes challenging, influences on the profession.

The growth in popularity of online therapy during the pandemic and beyond isn't just about its accessibility, it's about sheer client preference. Imagine spending the half hour before a therapy session relaxing in meditation or preparing a post-therapy meal, instead of sitting in the waiting room of an office and trying not to make eye contact with anyone. When able to focus through the eyes of a patient, part of what online therapy can offer is mere convenience and much more comfort – and is hugely valuable.

People interested in online therapy can now choose from therapists anywhere in the country, as opposed to being limited by where they live or work. They can browse profiles of potential therapists and easily make contact before committing to a course of treatment. Similarly, therapists may now attract clients from anywhere in the country, or internationally, bolstering their practice.

With a larger pool of therapists to choose from, clients now have greater control over how their treatment progresses. If the therapeutic match isn't working out, the client has options – and the clinician is likely to have a broader bank of referrals so a client can find the right match. This is mostly thanks to online therapist databases. Therapist/client matches can now be made based on genuine fit and clinician specialisation, not just whether the two live nearby.

In all, online therapy has proven to offer the capacity to greatly improve the accessibility of mental health treatment. With no need to travel, take time off from their busy schedules, or battle other logistical hurdles to getting care, clients are flocking to virtual therapy in droves. Beyond its boom during the COVID-19 pandemic, online therapy is here to stay as a force for good. But in this desire for change, how have we accounted for the operation of these services, and this way of choosing, booking, and working with therapists? As the dust from the pandemic settles, all stakeholders in the virtual mental health field will need to work together to ensure the use of technology is safe for everyone involved. So, who will pave the way for safe cybertherapy?

Stakeholders

Clients and practitioners are the primary stakeholders in a therapeutic relationship, but bringing therapy into cyberspace widens the network. Video-hosting platforms, practice management software, therapist databases, or any other online service that collects and processes personal health data, are now liable parties in the relationship. But it doesn't stop there. 'Big tech' and the marketers to whom they sell have their hands in the pie as well. It's important to understand who these stakeholders are and the role they play in preventing risk and creating viable solutions when problems arise. This is also not a static landscape. The rate of change in software services is an aspect that is also challenging. We must consider the value of trust, and the erosion of quality, not just due to education or therapeutic skills, but to the lack of accountability that is possible without a framework to which ethical standards can be applied.

Clients

There's no doubt that clients are the primary stakeholders in online therapy dealings. It is their vulnerability, their secrets, their fears, and the deepest details of their personhood that makes up the data in question (Knibbs & Hibberd, 2020). When we talk about data processing, the data we refer to are the intimate details that make a person who they are. The data are not just data – they represent human beings. When things go awry, clients are the stakeholders with the most to lose. Clients' vulnerability in communicating and attending therapy with a practitioner must be addressed.

Clinicians

As clinicians, we vow to protect our clients' livelihoods. It is in our moral and legal code to ensure the therapeutic spaces and records we keep are handled with the utmost care and respect. It is a core tenet of our job and the foundation of a trusting therapeutic relationship.

Online therapy spaces must be safe in order to maintain the integrity of the therapist/client relationship. Effective treatment cannot take place if a client doesn't trust the practitioner. A therapist's professional reputation cannot withstand a lack of trust from their clients. The success of their practice is on the line. This extends to all forms of communication and online practice.

Software programs and service platforms

Software providers are responsible for building and maintaining trustworthy platforms. Their practices must ensure that sensitive data are securely processed and stored. Foremost, these companies conduct themselves to avoid costly lawsuits and fines. A mistake could cost them far more than a preventative security solution would. Conversely, ensuring they foster trust in their consumers (clients and clinicians alike) strengthens their authority in the market and opens avenues for business expansion in the future. Technology is undoubtedly the 'landlord' of digital practice and should be an area where a high degree of influence should be able to be brought to bear.

Big tech

Big tech companies collect data to improve their revenue model and make more money by selling user data to advertisers. They're in the business of data collection, so any website or online platform processing large amounts of consumer data is like a gold mine to them. As the Internet landscape quickly evolves and changes, so do questions about the responsibility of big tech to protect and secure the data they collect. They are rarely concerned with the business of therapy specifically. They may deliver encryption for transport and storage, but there are many other benefits available to them in the metadata of our transactions that are economically useful.

Marketers

Advertisers partnering with big tech to deliver targeted ads benefit by identifying users who may already be looking for or are in need of mental health information. Their stakes lie in the private information that is shared through online therapy platforms and software. It's in advertisers' best interests to have as much data as possible to inform their campaigns. And while this poses clear ethical and legal issues in the context of client mental health data, some also argue that the ability to create relevant targeted marketing helps increase access to services and programs for those who need them (Palmer et al., 2022).

Information commissioner's office

The Information Commissioner's Office (ICO) is tasked with ensuring that personal information is processed and maintained in accordance with the Data Protection Act (DPA, 2018), and the General Data Protection Regulation of 2018. If a company or individual does not comply with these regulations, the ICO may enact fines or legal consequences. The ICO's stakes are in its legal responsibility to ensure Internet users' protected data remains protected.

In order to protect the information of a therapy client adequately, all stakeholders must work together to ensure the necessary precautions are in place and that the accountable parties abide by them. However, each stakeholder is operating on the principle of their own best interest. While money, career prospects, and reputation are on the line for most of the above stakeholders, these aspects cannot take precedence over the impact a data breach can have on the primary stakeholder: the therapy client.

Risks and impact

With the number of cyberattacks on the rise in recent years, it is wise to be wary of the risks of online therapy. Client data can be obtained by cybercriminals or simply misused by the middlemen in charge of telehealth platforms and online therapy tools. The impacts on clients and clinicians can range from invasive to downright devastating.

Many don't realise that data isn't just collected in the form of words typed and buttons clicked. Video and audio are data, too. It's not a given that the video platform you're using for your therapy sessions has the necessary protections for the sensitive data collected in an online session. If the platform isn't GDPR-compliant, you may as well be conducting therapy in a public park. But in this park, any number of criminals might be lurking in the shadows hoping to hear something they can steal from you or use against you.

Cybercriminals, a.k.a. 'hackers', make it their job to access private information or break into networks they're not meant to access. In 2020, hackers stole the therapy records of over 40,000 individuals in Finland (Knibbs & Hibberd, 2020). They emailed the clients 'demanding £180 in bitcoin or they would release the highly sensitive materials to friends and family'.

Not only does such an event cause significant distress for the clients whose information was leaked, but it also puts the company whose networks were compromised in the middle of hefty lawsuits. In this case, the company was looking at fines of up to £20 million and lawsuits from up to 40,000 affected clients. In the event that such a situation occurs in your practice, the person in the middle of those hefty lawsuits would be you.

Malicious hacking isn't the only source of a data breach. A data breach is any 'breach of security which leads to the accidental or unlawful destruction, loss, alteration, unauthorized disclosure of, or access to, personal data' (Knibbs & Hibberd, 2020). Examples of this as a private practitioner may include forgetting to log out of a computer to which someone else gained access, leaving the office unlocked and your hardware being stolen, or unknowingly having spyware on your computer.

Data breaches can also happen when the practice management (software, program, or website) has too many cooks in the kitchen, so to speak. Telehealth companies and directories are prime examples of companies that act as middlemen between therapists and their clients. These companies are not necessarily bound by the same privacy regulations as therapists and are often the source of private information leaks.

In a 2022 investigation conducted by Stat (a US health-oriented new website) and The Markup (a US non-profit news publication), 50 direct-to-consumer telehealth companies were analysed through the use of dummy accounts and testing to determine the extent to which these companies tracked and leaked sensitive user information (Palmer et al., 2022). These telehealth companies operate by collecting information via client-report intakes, then passing the intakes on to entities covered by the HIPAA, the United States law protecting sensitive patient health information. However, when telehealth companies act as middlemen, they themselves are under no obligation to comply with HIPAA – so, at the time of intake, clients are guaranteed no protection of their data whatsoever.

Though telehealth companies that operate in this way may make it known in their privacy policies, such documents can be hard for users to understand. Privacy policies and the use of trackers can change at any given time. And, to add to the deceit, the Stat investigation showed that 12 of the 50 companies advertised themselves to clients and clinicians as 'HIPAA-compliant'.

As previously mentioned, big tech companies run trackers on such sites to gather data to sell to advertisers. This data can include word-for-word answers to intake questions, users' names, email addresses, phone numbers, and more. In my own experience, I have seen the distressed words of a help-seeking client used verbatim as marketing copy in ad campaigns. Not only is this kind of invasion of privacy unethical, it also calls into question the competency of a copywriter or marketing manager to create trauma-informed, clinically sound recruitment content based on the data they collect.

Consider this example. If a client struggling with depressive symptoms sees enough targeted ads for antidepressants recommended by other patients, the client might feel pressured into taking something they don't actually need. A client might find they are spammed by marketers trying to sell mental health products or solutions that have nothing to do with the client's treatment, but are related to things their therapist knows or data their therapist has on the backend.

Even a private practitioner who works independently of telehealth directories must be wary of how they store data that they use to send clients promotional emails or newsletters. And on the side of the therapist, entering their personal information, such as a mobile number, into therapist databases is subject to the same tracking risks outlined above. You and your client both may be at risk for identity theft and fraud should personal identifying information from one of these directories be leaked.

In the event of a data breach in your private practice, you may be subject to monetary fines from the ICO, warnings, or bans on data processing (Knibbs & Hibberd, 2020). Such a ban could make it all but impossible to carry on with business as usual, as all sessions and documentation would need to return to in-person and hard-copy formats. Bans on data processing may be temporary or permanent and may include the erasure of all existing data.

The biggest risk, however, may be to your professional reputation. After a data breach, it's not unlikely that you would lose existing clients or be unable to acquire new clients as a result of the break in trust. Clients may seek compensation for damages, adding legal costs to the existing burden of any fines you may be subject to through the ICO.

The loss of a vocational reputation is large – but the loss of a personal reputation is massive. Clients made victims of a data breach risk discrimination, identity theft, fraud, distress, the loss of rights and freedoms, and even personal danger. Clients who share an underprivileged or minority sexual orientation, gender identity, religious affiliation, mental health status, or disability status with their therapist through an intake form or during a session risk this data being used against them. Should the information be made public, the individual could face harassment, threats, discrimination at work, job loss, loss of access to housing, or targeted violence.

Should data about personal relationships surface, as in the case of the Finland leak, clients may face irreparable ruptures in the trust of those relationships. In severe cases, such as clients suffering from domestic violence, the exposure of a client's therapeutic relationship or disclosure of abuse could put said client in danger of violence or death.

Needless to say, the impact of security risks on all stakeholders, especially clients, is profound. Despite its many benefits, online therapy as we know it today still has many safety gaps to be filled through education, regulation, and accountability. The largest gap, as evidenced by the above information, lies in the digital space between therapist and client – and the tech-related entities that reach and compete for user data therein.

Ethical solutions in tech

As we look at the future of online therapy, we must accept the fact of our current circumstances: the client/therapist relationship now involves more people than just the client and the therapist. Now that tech companies have inserted themselves between therapists and clients in the virtual world, are those companies prepared to take on the responsibilities of such an ethically and morally profound role? Are our regulatory bodies prepared to hold these parties accountable for how they use the data they collect? And are we as consumers prepared to sprint alongside tech companies whose mottoes are to 'move fast and break things?'.

As of now, the stakeholders involved don't yet understand one another. The Internet is relatively new, and online therapy is even newer. Tech companies leading the way and exercising power know little about what it means to uphold the integrity of a therapeutic relationship. And therapists will have gone through years of training and licensure not expecting to need to understand the ins and outs of cybersecurity or data mining. Marketing teams may not understand privacy regulations, and legal teams may not understand marketing strategies (Palmer et al., 2022). And clients, even as the primary stakeholders of the goings-on, may not have an understanding of any of the above.

Until we fully understand our roles and responsibilities in this innovative network, there will be a constant passing of the buck. Big tech claims it's the responsibility of advertisers not to use private information in their advertising. Legal experts believe tech companies should be accountable because of their power to 'vacuum up every ounce of personal data on the Internet' (Palmer et al., 2022).

Is it possible big tech does understand the personal risks of their users, and simply doesn't care? 'Even when it may seem that Big Tech is putting user data privacy first, it is usually about them lining their own pockets – again' (Chavez et al., 2022).

Privacy measures from Google that appear to be for the benefit of the public may actually be strategic moves to get an advantage over competitors or put blocks on other websites' abilities to track and collect data.

So, what are the actual rules and regulations in place for these tech companies and the advertisers they partner with? They're left up to a region's supervisory authority. In the UK, that authority is the ICO. Currently, the DPA and GDPR are in place to protect user information. But just like tech companies can skirt HIPAA, they may skirt GDPR if they're not based in the UK.

In 2019, Google was fined €50 million for 'lack of transparency, inadequate information and lack of valid consent regarding the ads personalization' (European Data Protection Board, 2019). The ICO also keeps a list of its most recent enforcement actions available for the public to view on its website. But for a supervisory authority to take disciplinary action, it first must become aware of the breach from a concerned third party. As consumers who embody that third party, how much attention are we really paying to our cyber privacy? Should a data breach arise, would we even know – or care?

As a society, we've become accustomed to handing over our personal information on the Internet. Perhaps this began with ignorance and a lack of understanding of how easily accessible our data was to others. But with attention-grabbing headlines about data breaches in the news almost daily, we can no longer claim ignorance. We sign up for new accounts and apps with little to no hesitation, agreeing to terms of service without bothering to read through them. We seem resigned to the idea that companies already know everything about us anyway, so 'What can we do about it?'.

Despite hearing about the backlash and lawsuits big tech companies are facing, we are yet to see a significant change in how those companies operate. And although the public sentiment is generally complacent, there are entities taking steps to make a change. Even though our supervisory authorities seem slow to lay down the laws, initiatives such as The Ethical Tech Project are paving the way for a safer future. At the time of the writing of this chapter, The Ethical Tech Project is organising to convene 'businesses, academics, and governments to build standards for the use of data in technology' (The Ethical Tech Project, n.d.).

As private practitioners in the online therapy world, where do we fall among the crowd? Are we complacent, or fighting for ethical data collection? Until we see a change in policy and accountability for how big tech manages our personal data, we must be the latter. As clinicians, we need to be aware of the path our clients' data takes before it reaches us, and where it will be for the seven years (in most cases) that we need to store it. This means acknowledging the problem. We advocate for our clients' welfare in their presenting issues, to remove barriers to access to care, and for the integrity of our profession. Now, we must also advocate for our clients' data privacy, and in doing so, set the new standard.

Doing our part

Cybersecurity is becoming part of your role as a therapist. And it's not just your moral duty – it's the law. Any time you conduct an online therapy session or use the Internet for documentation, you're processing client data. In the terms of the GDPR, this makes you a 'processor': any individual responsible for the processing of data belonging to a UK citizen (Knibbs & Hibberd, 2020).

As a business owner, you're also considered what the GDPR calls a data 'controller'. A controller is an entity that determines how processed data is collected, stored, and used. The controller is not your IT professional or big tech. As a business owner in private practice, *it is you*.

You may wonder how or why you would be the target of a cyberattack or data breach, as you're only one solo practitioner. Who would bother to target one clinician with 20 clients? But even small businesses like yours are vulnerable, especially if you're not utilising your energy and resources for security. This can be intimidating and, now that you know the risks involved, you might be afraid to host an online practice. Yes, there's much outside of your control that could go wrong. But there are things you can do to protect your business and your clients.

The first, and most important, is to educate yourself. Reading books like this one is a great start. Though it can be hard to stay on top of all the shifts taking place in the tech world, keeping updated with the latest reported breaches, changes in policies, and best practices, can save you a headache later on.

Second, educate your clients. It is the responsibility of the ICO to educate institutions on data protection practices. But are your clients educated? Many of them may not think twice about the risks they're taking when they consent to online treatment with you. Your clients should be able to trust you in all facets of how you conduct business with them. Provide in your informed consent 'an intelligible and easily accessible form, using clear and plain language [that] should not contain unfair terms' (Knibbs & Hibberd, 2020). This can take the form of a privacy notice on your website or as a privacy policy in your contract.

The Essential Guide for Therapists for Protection of Data (Knibbs & Hibberd, 2020), offers more suggestions for documents that should be essential to any online practice. These include an information security and data protection policy, an acceptable use policy, an incident management and data breach process, a privacy and cookie policy, an IT operations protection process, a subject access request (SAR) Process, a data privacy impact assessment (DPIA), and a records of processing activities (RoPA). Necessary protection procedures recommended in *The Essential Guide* include malware protection, a virtual private network (VPN), patch management, encryption, website security, and backups.

In the same way that you put care and attention into your physical therapy room, you should put care and attention into your virtual therapy room. There are steps you can take to increase your client's comfort and let them know you respect their privacy. When using a video platform to conduct a session, use passwords or codes as frequently as possible to limit access to the meeting. You can enable a 'waiting room' in the meeting whereby attendees must be manually permitted to have access to the meeting. This creates a two-step process for entry, as if your client had to walk through two locked doors before reaching your 'office'. The video platform you use may also provide an option to 'lock' the session once it has begun. It may also be appropriate to educate your client about their own best practices while attending video sessions. Encouraging your client to call in from a private location is not only in the best interest of your client but also of your practice.

Another aspect to consider when conducting video sessions is the background of your or your client's screens. As mentioned above, all audio and video are data. It's prudent to remove personal belongings such as family photos or confidential information such as documents on a desk, as this information will be processed along with everything else (Knibbs & Hibberd, 2020).

In the event that you need to record a session for supervision purposes (or any other purpose), you must ask your client for consent, providing an explanation so the consent can be informed. *The Essential Guide* outlines the need to ask for consent before recording and verbally confirm the client's consent to record once you have begun recording and before you continue with your session. Any recordings should be protected through adequate security measures like the ones listed above and destroyed when no longer needed.

It takes time, care, and financial investment to ensure your private practice remains protected from cybercrime and data misuse. However, the inconveniences and monetary costs are a small price to pay for the integrity of your practice, your clients' safety, and your own livelihood and career. The regular expenses of GDPR-compliant software and protection products are minuscule compared to a fine from the ICO or lawsuits from your clients.

We cannot deny the leadership void in the industry at this time. But with it rapidly evolving, and with diligence from legislator, individual clinicians like you, and groups like The Ethical Tech Project, software providers and big tech will be forced to update their products to meet the demands of GDPR, HIPAA, and users. Currently, we have to deal with an unstable and precarious landscape in the online therapy world. But the advantages of online therapy are astronomical for the future of accessible mental healthcare. There *is* a future in which online therapy is safe and ethical for all. Until then, stay tuned into the progress and keep fighting for your clients' safety through security practices and advocacy. Your small acts of power make an impact.

References

Anthony, K., & Nagel, D.M. (2010). *Therapy Online: A Practical Guide*. London: Sage Publications, 64.

BACP. (2021). *BACP Mindometer Report 2021*. BACP. Retrieved 2022, from https://www.bacp.co.uk/media/12065/bacp-mindometer-report-2021.pdf.

Chavez, T., Johnson, M., & Andersen, J. (2022, 28 February). We need common-sense privacy regulation to curb Big Tech. *Fortune*. Retrieved 16 December 2022, from https://fortune.com/2022/02/28/data-privacy-regulation-consumer-demands-big-tech/.

Data Protection Act (2018). https://www.legislation.gov.uk/ukpga/2018/12/contents/enacted.

The Ethical Tech Project (n.d.). Building the infrastructure for ethical tech. Retrieved 16 December 2022, from https://www.ethicaltechproject.com/.

European Data Protection Board. (2019, 21 January). The CNIL's Restricted Committee imposes a financial penalty of 50 million euros against Google LLC. Retrieved 16 December 2022, from https://edpb.europa.eu/news/national-news/2019/cnils-restricted-committee-imposes-financial-penalty-50-million-euros_en.

GDPR (2018). https://gdpr-info.eu/.

GDPR (UK) (2020). https://ico.org.uk/for-organisations/data-protection-and-the-eu/data-protection-and-the-eu-in-detail/the-uk-gdpr/.

Knibbs, C., & Hibberd, G. (2020). *The Essential Guide for Therapists to Protection of Data*. Available at www.privacy4.co.uk.

Litam, S.D.A., Ausloos, C.D., & Harrichand, J.J.S. (2021). Stress and resilience among professional counselors during the COVID-19 Pandemic, *Journal of Counseling & Development, 99*(4): 384–395.

Palmer, K., Feathers, T., & Fondrie-Teitler, S. (2022, 13 December). 'Out of control': Dozens of telehealth startups sent sensitive health information to big tech companies. STAT. Retrieved 16 December 2022, from https://www.statnews.com/2022/12/13/telehealth-facebook-google-tracking-health-data/.

Rauch, J. (2018, 28 September). The history of online therapy. Talkspace. Retrieved 16 December 2022, from https://www.talkspace.com/blog/history-online-therapy/.

Situmorang, D.D.B. (2020, October). Online/cyber counseling services in the COVID-19 outbreak: Are they really new? *The Journal of Pastoral Care & Counseling*. Retrieved 16 December 2022, from https://www.ncbi.nlm.nih.gov/pmc/articles/PMC7528539/#sec6-1542305020948170title.

Statista Research Department. (2022, 18 October). Internet usage in the UK. Retrieved 16 December 2022, from https://www.statista.com/topics/3246/Internet-usage-in-the-uk/#topicHeader__wrapper.

Weinberg, H., Leighton, A., & Rolnick, A. (2022) *Advances in Online Therapy: Emergence of a New Paradigm*. Abingdon: Taylor & Francis.

Worley-James, S. (2022). *Online Counselling: An Essential Guide*. Monmouth: PCCS Books, 46.

Young, D., & Edwards, E. (2020, 6 May). Telehealth and disability: Challenges and opportunities for care. National Health Law Program. Retrieved 16 December 2022, from https://healthlaw.org/telehealth-and-disability-challenges-and-opportunities-for-care/.

8 Online professionalism

Rory Lees-Oakes

Introduction

The social media minefield.

It would seem that not a week passes without the press publishing details of embarrassing or inappropriate social media posts attributed to someone in the public eye.

In 2019 an article in the UK-based *Metro* newspaper (Mann, 2019) ran an article about Labour member of parliament, Naz Shah, who in 2017 liked and retweeted a Twitter post that strongly intimated that the victims who were abused by a grooming gang in the town of Rotherham in the UK, should stay quiet for the sake of diversity.

Shah later deleted the retweet and, according to the newspaper report, tried to mitigate her actions by stating: 'This was a genuine accident eight days ago that was rectified within minutes. To suggest otherwise is absolute nonsense.'

In 2021, the UK-based *Independent* newspaper (Ritschel, 2021) ran an article about Alexi McCammond, the 27-year-old, newly appointed editor of *Teenage Vogue*, who resigned after a series of racist tweets she had written as a teenager resurfaced.

Commenting on Twitter after her resignation, McCammond reflected that her '*past tweets have overshadowed the work I've done*'.

The current zeitgeist of naming and shaming those who transgress on social media is summarised as *Tweet in haste, repent at leisure.* This maxim applies to those in the public eye and those who practise in the psychotherapeutic professions.

The importance of social media professionalism

What you see is what you get.

Throughout the history of psychotherapy, from its earliest theorists to students currently in training, the discipline has been characterised by compassion and service to those who find themselves in emotional distress.

Members of the public seeking psychotherapeutic help must have an unbiased view of the profession. Any obstacle put in the way of a potential client accessing support could sometimes become a matter of life or death.

DOI: 10.4324/9781003364184-9

Membership bodies have, through the years, developed ethical frameworks and best practice resources in several areas, especially around confidentiality, yet the same organisations have, in the author's experience, been relatively slow to respond with guidance to a growing tendency of misuse of social media by some practitioners in the psychotherapeutic profession.

Thankfully, leading UK membership/ethical bodies have caught up and have now stated their expectations on how members should use social media given the potential impact disinhibited social media (see Suler, 2004) use may have on public confidence in the profession.

The British Association of Counselling and Psychotherapy (BACP), a UK-based membership/ethical body, has published guidance for its members and clarified in what circumstances they may enact a misconduct process, stating:

> Our professional conduct process focuses primarily on serious concerns where there's a public risk or where public confidence in the professions could be undermined by one of our member's actions.
>
> (BACP, n.d.)

Another leading UK membership/ethical body, National Counselling and Psychotherapy Society (NCPS), has been even more granular in its guidance to practitioners, offering the following observation in a resource available in the member's section of their website titled 'Communication Guidance':

> Whether we identify ourselves as a counsellor and/or psychotherapist on our profile, we should act responsibly at all times and uphold the profession's reputation. It goes without saying that it is a serious breach of our ethical code to discuss client or work-related issues online in any non-secure, unencrypted medium. Publishing pictures of clients or service users online is completely prohibited.
>
> (NCPS, 2022)

UK membership/ethical bodies are not the only professional bodies concerned about how disinhibited social media use may impact public confidence in the psychotherapeutic profession (see Suler, 2004).

An article in the *New York Times* titled 'Psychologist Jordan Peterson could lose license if he refuses social media "re-education"' (Reilly, 2023) outlines how the controversial Canadian psychologist Dr Jordan Peterson has been directed by his licencing body, The College of Psychologists of Ontario, to undertake social media re-education for what the article describes as 'comments he made on Twitter and the Joe Rogan podcast'.

At the time of writing, Dr Peterson is forming a legal response to his licencing body and strongly refutes the need for social media re-education.

In conclusion, UK membership/ethical bodies[1] are actively developing codes of ethics and guidance on their members' acceptable use of social media.

As an act of reflective and deliberate practice, practitioners should review ethical guidance on the acceptable use of social media. Clinical supervisors may point supervisees to this guidance as formative continuing professional development (CPD) opportunity.

A complaint about a practitioner's inappropriate comments or breaking of confidentiality on social media would almost certainly be referenced against current ethical guidelines on the misuse of social media.

Factors contributing to the misuse of social media

'Facebook Groups to provide users more control' is the headline of an article published by the *Guardian* newspaper online in October 2010. Charles Arthur, the now former technology editor of the newspaper, reflected, 'Facebook has launched "groups" – its attempt to mirror the way that people interact in the real world, where we interact with small groups of people such as family, work colleagues and wider friends, rather than everyone at once' (Arthur, 2010).

Anyone who has been a member of a Facebook or social media group may raise an eyebrow at the suggestion that they 'mirror the way that people interact in the real world'.

The majority of social media interactions are helpful and supportive, but there is also a tendency for some interactions to become controversial, toxic, threatening, and, in some cases, illegal.

In 2022 the UK-based Crown Prosecution Service (CPS) published details of the successful prosecution of a 27-year-old man under Section 127 of the Communications Act. The article described the offence as 'sending by a public communication an offensive and menacing message' (CPS, 2022). The person in question had posted a racist, hateful comment on a local Facebook Group.

So, what factors contribute to the members of some groups posting racist, homophobic, misogynistic, transphobic, and, in some cases, threatening responses and content?

What makes some therapists behave differently online from in face-to-face interactions?

From a psychological perspective, John Suler, PhD, Professor of Psychology at Ryder University in the United States, outlined a plausible hypothesis: 'the disinhibition effect'.

His 2004 research paper titled 'The online disinhibition effect' (Suler, 2004) outlined six factors that interact with each other creating the online disinhibition effect: dissociative anonymity, invisibility, asynchronicity, solipsistic introjection, dissociative imagination, and minimisation of authority.

According to the research, some individuals psychologically distance themselves from the people they interact with online. Those who adopt this phenomenological position come to believe that they are anonymous, the rules of social engagement do not apply, that communication with others is a form of a game, and, at any time, they can run away by logging out and logging off.

Hence the term 'keyboard warrior' denotes a person who makes abusive or aggressive posts on the Internet, concealing their true identity and believing that they are not accountable for what they write or say.

Another contributing factor may be the ongoing societal debate on what constitutes free speech.

Social media platforms such as Twitter and Meta (formerly known as Facebook) have become the default public square where individuals debate matters that concern them.

While some users believe they are entitled to freedom of expression and debate without censorship, others argue that 'hate speech' is unacceptable and 'free speech has consequences'.

A mixture of disinhibition and an ongoing debate about what constitutes 'free speech' can lead therapists to engage in questionable or even unethical online behaviour.

Some examples of questionable and unethical online behaviour

In 2010, Facebook launched 'groups', a place to connect, learn, and meet with people who share similar interests. One can create or join a *group* for anything — from baking to astrophysics. There is almost certainly a group to support anyone's specific interest or profession.

A cursory search of Facebook using the term 'counselling' or 'psychotherapy' will return many groups offering support to qualified practitioners and students in training.

It is possible to categorise some groups as generic, such as the author's own Facebook group 'Counselling Tutor', which allows members to debate various psychotherapeutic topics and is open to anyone practising or studying counselling or psychotherapy.

Other groups have a more specific remit. For example, 'Counsellors Together', a UK-based group whose 'About' page states: 'A group for UK-based counsellors interested in working together to end the culture and prevalence of unpaid work within our profession.' The group also offers support and restorative activities for its members.

Some groups appeal to a specific demographic, such as the Network for Younger Counsellors and Psychotherapists (NYCP). This UK-based group's mission statement states: 'NYCP is a relational and collaborative platform to empower, connect and resource younger counsellors and psychotherapists' (NYCP, n.d.).

One thing all these groups have in common (the author is a member of all of them) is that they are well moderated and have entry criteria in the form of questions potential members have to fill in before being accepted into the group.

They are also closed groups, meaning only group members can view postings or discussion threads and they have group rules which members have to agree to before being allowed entry.

To a great degree, the groups are self-moderating. Members alert group administrators and moderators to postings that break the group's guidelines or may bring the profession into disrepute.

Group administrators have at their disposal the use of automated tools (Meta Platforms, Inc., n.d.) that Facebook provides to remove or flag content that may be offensive or controversial. However, inappropriate postings may still occur even with the most robust moderation and filtering.

A mixture of disinhibition and a misjudged idea that a closed Facebook group is a 'safe space' can lead practitioners to engage in professionally questionable behaviour, especially around areas of confidentiality. For example, therapists who use the group as pseudo-supervisors may post questions such as 'I have a client who is suicidal, what should I do?' or 'My client is using drugs. Any advice about interventions?.

Besides the danger of asking advice from people one has never met and whose qualifications and experience in psychotherapy are taken for granted, there is also the question of confidentiality.

Therapeutic voyeurism

Some therapists anonymously search the social media profiles of their clients to assuage their curiosity or, more worryingly, to garner information about their client's life in the misguided belief that the newly found knowledge may somehow aid the therapeutic process.

A therapist can quickly disadvantage a client by reflecting back information the client has not disclosed. The impact of therapeutic voyeurism is that boundaries become blurred or collapse completely as the client picks up that the therapist knows more about them than they have disclosed. This behaviour demonstrates a total disregard for the ethical principle of beneficence and can potentially create a toxic power imbalance.

The author knows of one complaint a UK ethical body upheld where the therapist viewed their client's LinkedIn profile. Unfortunately for the therapist, LinkedIn displays to their members the names of those who have viewed their profile, which meant the client could tell the therapist had looked them up.

In response to the client's enquiry into this intrusion, the therapist replied: 'This is what therapists do.' Unsurprisingly, the ethics board upheld the complaint and imposed a sanction. One can only speculate if the client continued their therapy with another therapist.

Catfishing

Unlike practitioners, clients do not have any obligations under an ethical framework and may search social media for their therapist. The question is, what will they find?

What is the therapist's favourite football team or band? Political affiliation? Faith position? What about pictures of family and friends? Or their partner? Children? Grandchildren? Home? Holiday pictures of their therapist in swimwear or *au naturel*?

An open social media profile may leave the therapist susceptible to a worryingly new phenomenon of online abuse called 'catfishing'.

An online behaviour outlined in a research paper titled 'Adult attachment and online dating deception: A theory modernized' (Mosley et al., 2020) as: 'An extreme form of online dating deception, also known as "catfishing," involves falsely representing oneself to a potential romantic partner, without the intention of meeting in person.'

Social media companies have made considerable efforts to delete fake profiles, but people still create them. The danger of 'catfishing' is that the therapist may receive unsolicited romantic or sexual approaches or friendship requests from individuals who hide their identities.

Social media boundaries and client confidence

Without labouring the point, a client having unrestricted access to their therapist's social media account may have unintended consequences. For clients who experience difficulty with self-regulation or attachment, this could lead to boundary fractures, such as contacting the therapist directly via social media or commenting in session on aspects of the therapist's private life.

Shawn Ryan, a YouTuber and former special forces operative, commented on this phenomenon in a video titled 'Finding the Right Therapist – 5 Tips from a Navy SEAL' (Ryan, 2020). Ryan was outlining to his military audience steps to understanding how to engage with therapy for PTSD. Ryan observed that seeing a picture of his therapist in a bikini (he used the colloquialism 'string') may cause him unwanted distractions and attraction – the underlying message of possible erotic or eroticised countertransference is clear.

Sometimes, a client may take offence at the therapist's political position. The author has seen two social media posts from therapists asking: 'Why would you visit a Tory voting therapist?'[2] or 'What kind of therapist votes Labour?'[3]. In contrast, the client may see the therapist as a 'fellow traveller', leading to the therapist pushing the boundaries of relevant self-disclosure.

For the above reasons, many practitioners use a 'nom de plume' on their social media accounts, activate the privacy settings, and remove any identifying images.

There are excellent examples of online professionalism, from therapists who advertise their services on social media to politically and socially underrepresented and excluded groups. Their messaging acknowledges inclusivity instead of engaging in disinhibited polemic and ad hominem attacks.

Online professionalism – good practice

In light of the potential pitfalls of using social media as a professional, let us explore some areas of good practice.

Security settings

Those with social media accounts may find the following observations on basic security helpful.

- Many therapists change their names on social media profiles and remove any identifying profile images to avoid clients searching for them.
- It is also helpful to visit the security settings on Facebook profiles to restrict access to viewing posts and images on the timeline to those one specifically nominates.
- Users should avoid using easy-to-guess passwords, such as 12345678, when choosing a password for their social media accounts.

Online privacy

Social media applications such as Facebook sometimes use a smartphone's GPS feature to track users' locations. In some cases, this information is posted in the body of posts or tagged into photographs, thus identifying the user's location.

Users may wish to remove the location feature in their social media accounts by denying applications such as Facebook, LinkedIn, and Twitter access to the phone's GPS function. Users who need help switching off the GPS settings for social media can find this information on the phone manufacturer's websites.

Facebook helpfully provides online resources – 'Use our security features, such as login alerts and approvals, and review and update your security settings at any time' (Meta, 2023) – which assist users in reviewing and updating their security settings.

Developing a professional presence online

For those therapists who wish to use social media to promote their practice, the way forward may be to set up a business page, opening a social media business account can have several advantages, including:

1 **Increased visibility:** Social media platforms are popular and widely used, so creating a business account can increase therapist visibility to potential clients searching for therapy services.
2 **Establishing a professional online presence:** A social media business account can help a therapist establish a professional online presence to enhance their reputation.
3 **Building trust with potential clients:** Sharing informative and educational content on professional social media accounts can help build trust with potential clients, which can be important when they are seeking therapy services.
4 **Sharing resources and information:** When related to mental health, shared resources and information can benefit clients and other professionals.
5 **Improving engagement with clients:** Social media provides a platform to engage with clients and answer their questions about therapy or mental health concerns.
6 **Networking with other mental health professionals:** Social media can be used to connect and network with other mental health professionals, which can be helpful for referrals or professional development opportunities.

By creating a professional/business profile, therapists can control their online presence and set a professional boundary for clients regarding contact details and availability.

Conclusion

As a result of social media, human communication has changed significantly. Ideas, images, and even our identities can now travel worldwide in milliseconds.

Consequently, those who 'tweet/post in haste' may find themselves repenting not at leisure but in front of an ethics panel or explaining themselves to their peers.

Being reflective and reflexive around social media presence should be considered an act of self-care, self-compassion, and professional probity.

Sharma and Kharas (2017) share a valid observation from Erin Bury, a former technology journalist, entrepreneur, and expert in social media communication, who wryly observes:

> *Don't say anything online that you wouldn't want plastered on a billboard with your face on it.*

An apt parable for the epoch of social media and for those therapists who navigate its many minefields

Notes

1 This term is used to highlight the voluntary nature of membership of an ethical body in the absence of UK government regulation at the time of writing.
2 'Tory' is a colloquial term for someone who votes for or is a member of the UK Conservative Party, which historically is on the right of the political spectrum.
3 Labour is the name of a UK political party, historically on the left of the political spectrum.

References

Arthur, C. (2010, 7 October). Facebook groups to offer users more control. *The Guardian*. Retrieved 3 February 2023, from https://www.theguardian.com/technology/2010/oct/07/facebook-groups.

BACP (n.d.). Guidance on the use of social media information for members. Retrieved 1 February 2023, from https://www.bacp.co.uk/membership/membership-policies/social-media/.

CPS (2022, 23 March). Hate crime. Retrieved 3 February 2023, from https://www.cps.gov.uk/mersey-cheshire/news/hate-online-crime.

Mann, T. (2019, 12 December). MP shares tweet saying abuse victims should 'shut their mouths'. *Metro*. Retrieved 31 January 2023, from https://metro.co.uk/2017/08/23/mp-shares-tweet-saying-abuse-victims-should-shut-their-mouths-for-good-of-diversity-6872181/.

Meta Platforms, Inc. (n.d.). Moderation. Meta Business Help Center. Retrieved 6 February 2023, from https://www.facebook.com/business/help/1323914937703529.

Mosley, M.A., Lancaster, M., Parker, M.L., & Campbell, K. (2020). Adult attachment and online dating deception: A theory modernized. *Sexual and Relationship Therapy, 35*(2), 227–243. https://doi.org/10.1080/14681994.2020.1714577.

NCPS (2022, 1 February). Social networking media (Facebook, LinkedIn, Twitter, etc.). Retrieved 1 February 2023, from https://nationalcounsellingsociety.org/about-us/code-of-ethics.

NYCP (n.d.). Home [Facebook page]. Facebook. Retrieved 8 February 2023, from https://www.facebook.com/groups/1454766688043600.

Reilly, P. (2023, 6 January). Psychologist Jordan Peterson could lose license if he refuses social media 're-education'. *New York Post.* Retrieved 1 February 2023, from https://nypost.com/2023/01/05/jordan-peterson-could-lose-psychologist-license-if-he-refuses-social-media-re-education/.

Ritschel, C. (2021, 19 March). The tweets that cost former Teen Vogue editor Alexi McCammond her job. *The Independent.* Retrieved 31 January 2023, from https://www.independent.co.uk/life-style/alexi-mccammond-tweets-teen-vogue-editor-resign-b1819768.html.

Ryan, S. (2019) Finding the Right Therapist – 5 Tips from a Navy SEAL (video). Vigilance Elite. Available at https://www.youtube.com/watch?v=FBoe9D2DlZg. Accessed: 12 February 2023.

Sharma, V., & Kharas, H. (2017). Execution. In The Indestructible Brand: Crisis Management in the Age of Social Media. Sage, p. 26.

Suler, J. (2004). The online disinhibition effect. *Cyberpsychology & Behavior: The Impact of the Internet, Multimedia and Virtual Reality on Behavior and Society, 7*(3), 321–326. https://doi.org/10.1089/1094931041291295.

Social media

Counselling Tutor (n.d.). Home [Facebook page]. Facebook. Retrieved 8 February 2023, from https://www.facebook.com/groups/472203952972076.

Counsellors Together (n.d.). Home [Facebook page]. Facebook. Retrieved 8 February 2023, from https://www.facebook.com/groups/counsellorstogetheruk.

Security Features and Tips (n.d.). Facebook Help Centre [Facebook page]. Facebook. Retrieved 12 February 2023, from https://www.facebook.com/help/285695718429403.

9 Data protection, children, and the law

Elizabeth Milovidov and Catherine Knibbs

Introduction

Educators, practitioners, and psychotherapists must not only protect the individual children that they are working with, but they must also protect the data of those same children. Data protection goes beyond just maintaining the confidentiality and respecting children's rights to privacy; data protection extends to data security and adherence to legal data requirements.

When working with children, educators, practitioners, and psychotherapists often collect and store sensitive information about a child's mental health, personal life, family issues, and experiences with the understanding that they will keep the information private and may only share it with others, when necessary, for safeguarding and other legal processes and with the appropriate consent. In the United Kingdom, the legislation surrounding this is *Working Together to Safeguard Children (2018)* and *Keeping Children safe in Education (2022)*.

However, the profession of counselling and psychotherapy must always balance confidentiality and safeguarding with the therapeutic alliance (the relationship between therapist and client/patient), unless lawful processes need to be reported, such as terrorism and crime. You can find out more about this ethical dilemma in the guidelines for your membership body, as this book is dedicated to the keeping, maintaining, and sharing of that information (known as data). Furthermore, here we are not looking to debate this ethical issue about when it is necessary to share data and for what purposes.

We are, rather, stating that educators, practitioners, and psychotherapists have a *role* in keeping children's data secure and respecting their rights to privacy. This includes being transparent about how they collect and use children's data, and only collecting and using data that is necessary and relevant to the work that they are doing with them. It is equally important that once data is collected and stored, educators, practitioners, and psychotherapists ensure the security of the data by using secure servers, encrypting data, and regularly updating security protocols to protect against data breaches or unauthorised access. Earlier chapters in this book guide you on how to do this.

DOI: 10.4324/9781003364184-10

Confidentiality and privacy

Confidentiality and privacy are essential considerations for educators, practitioners, and psychotherapists when treating children. Respecting a child's privacy rights and ensuring confidentiality means making certain that sensitive information about a child's mental health or personal life is not shared without the child's consent, except in cases where there is a legal obligation to do so (e.g. if a child is at risk of harm).[1] In the United Kingdom, English law provides that the overriding consideration is to safeguard the child (The Children Act 1989).[2]

It is the responsibility of educators, practitioners, and psychotherapists to keep this information private and to only share it with others when necessary and with the appropriate consent, such as sharing information with other professionals or agencies (for example, with a school counsellor or social worker) if it is deemed necessary for the wellbeing of the child. Maintaining confidentiality also means being mindful of the child's physical privacy (for example, ensuring that confidential conversations take place in private and that any written records are kept secure).

If a child is accessing counselling in a school setting, consideration must be given to the fact that children are often seen accessing the service by other children and adults in the school, or in some circumstances they may sign up for these services (on sheets of paper that can be seen by others), and due consideration must be given as to how a child may be granted the right to privacy in these circumstances. For example, a counsellor collecting a child from a classroom space may not provide this level of confidentiality or privacy. A way to approach the thinking behind this is to consider how you would feel as an adult if this was your experience of such a process. What if you had certain circumstances that you wanted to keep private and the knowledge of accessing these services brought questions about where you were going or why? Maintaining confidentiality and protecting the children's privacy helps build trust and rapport and is a key component of ethical practice.

Confidentiality and privacy protection go beyond organisational policies and colourful manifestos, but it must be extended to every possible scenario involving the child, as seen above with respect to note-taking, child collection, and more. Maintaining confidentiality and protection privacy are equally important from a legal standpoint, as violations of confidentiality and privacy can have serious consequences.

Distinctions and differences

A simple way to understand the difference between confidentiality and privacy is to remember that privacy concerns the person and confidentiality concerns the data.[3] Privacy is the right to be left alone or to be free from interference,[4] whereas confidentiality refers to the forms of the information that was shared. So, when you think of how a child may want to control access to their information, this refers to privacy:

- Methods used to set up a session.
- Methods used to note information during the session.

This is distinct from confidentiality, which could include:

- Any consent forms that you provide the child or family.
- Methods to retain and process the data gathered during the session.

Case study

> Mary is a child counsellor who recently suffered a broken leg while riding her horse. She contracted via the parent (Liam's mum in this case) to continue sessions with Liam over a video platform so that he didn't miss out on sessions while her leg healed. Liam's mum was keen for this to happen and emailed Mary with Liam's personal email address so that she could set up the appointments with him. Mary used her personal email account and let Liam know she would call him on Thursday at 4 pm when he got home from school for his counselling session. Liam used his phone on the way to school and back, and on the bus, he opened his emails while sitting next to Tom, who was shoulder surfing and reading his (Liam's) emails. Tom exclaimed to the rest of the children on the bus that Liam was seeing a counsellor called Mary Louise and that they had a website which he eagerly shared with the other occupants. Liam did not attend his session that evening; and when his mum came back from work, he was really angry with her for sharing his email with the counsellor without telling him. Liam is 14.

Questions

- Now you have read the earlier chapters do you think Mary or Liam's mum were in breach of Liam's privacy and confidentiality?
- What do you think happened when the other children got the name of the counsellor's website and what would happen to the data collection of the other children if she had Google analytics or tracking software installed on her website?

Data security

In addition to protecting the confidentiality of children's personal information, it is also important for educators, practitioners, and psychotherapists to ensure that the data they collect and store is secure. This may include measures such as using secure servers, encrypting data, and regularly updating security protocols. Again, this reflects a need for adequate training in this area.

Data security is also important in the event of a data breach, where sensitive information about a child is accidentally or intentionally accessed or disclosed without permission. It is essential that educators, practitioners, and psychotherapists have a plan in place for responding to a breach and that we take steps to minimise the risk of breaches occurring in the first place. This may include implementing robust security measures and regularly training staff on best practices for data security.

Case study

Giles is working in a primary school. He sees children in his office and takes paper notes for his supervision. He is careful not to write the child's name and so uses a number to maintain the confidentiality of the sessions. He is asked to write up some notes on the school system called CPOMS and when he is finished, he logs off for the day. Giles puts the notes into his bag and takes them home where he will write them up in a word document and store them on his computer at home. Giles has three children who have their own accounts on the computer. His files are backed up to iCloud and he has a document-sharing function enabled on the computer for family photos, files, and music.

Questions

- When you consider your practice, your business or where you are in charge of data controlling and processing, what systems do *you* have in place for adequately securing data, and do you have a cybersecurity policy and procedures in place for this?
- Are the systems you use backed up by certification, such as ISO 27001?
- Have you explained to each child in a language they can understand what you do with this data and how you protect it?
- Looking at the procedures Giles is following, as explained above, is Giles in breach of any data protection laws?
- (*Hints*: his paperwork is in his bag, how is this secured? Is it destroyed after typing it up? Can his children/family access these documents?)

Data retention and destruction

Educators, practitioners, and psychotherapists should also be aware of any regulations or guidelines related to how long they should keep data on children, and when and how they should destroy that data. Proper data retention and destruction practices help to protect the confidentiality and privacy of the children and are necessary to comply with relevant laws and regulations. It is important to retain this information for as long as necessary, as it may be needed to inform treatment approaches or to document progress. However, it is also important to be mindful of data retention periods and to destroy data once they are no longer needed.

Data retention and destruction practices may be governed by laws, regulations, or professional guidelines. For example, there may be specific requirements for how long certain types of data must be retained, or for how data should be securely destroyed when no longer needed. It is important for educators and psychotherapists to be familiar with these requirements and to follow them when retaining and destroying data about children.

In addition to complying with legal and professional guidelines, proper data retention and destruction practices are also important for protecting the confidentiality and privacy of children. Retaining data for longer than necessary or failing to securely destroy data can put children's personal information at risk of unauthorised access or disclosure.

Often insurance companies stipulate how long data should be kept.

The co-author (Catherine Knibbs) is aware of practices of child counselling services and member bodies keeping data for the lifetime of a child (beyond the age of 18 or 25 and until their death) on electronic systems, where the necessary part of this process seems to be outside of a 'reasonable' amount of time. Remember, that the longer you hold data the higher the likelihood of breaches, destruction, and decomposition.

How would you explain this to a child under 13, and over 13, and how would you gain appropriate consent given this long length of time? Is it possible to consent to a lifetime of data retention, other than for example the National Health Service (NHS) holding your medical records?

Case study

> Miriam is a practitioner in her late 60s. She is approaching retirement and she is slowing down her practice and winding up the cases she has with children to focus on adult work. She has decided that she will finish working with her patients by the age of 70, as she feels she can reasonably work until that age. Her membership body has requested that she follows her liability insurance for the data retention period and processes. Miriam's youngest client is 3 years old. Her insurance company states that she keeps children's data until 7 years past their 18th birthday.

Questions

- Is this a reasonable process for Miriam to engage with, as she is not very good with computers and keeps many of her notes on paper – though she has to contact the associate services she works for via email?
- Should she keep all the emails ever sent to and from the associate services as part of her obligations to the child, insurance company, or association service procedures, and what will Miriam need to do to keep up with the changing technology to ensure those emails are kept safe, secure, and not breached?

Data sharing and consent

In some cases, it may be necessary for educators, practitioners, and psychotherapists to share data about a child with other professionals or agencies, such as a school counsellor or a social worker. In these cases, it is important to get the consent of the child (or their parent or guardian) before sharing the data, and to share only the minimum amount of information necessary.

In some cases, it may also be necessary to share this information with other professionals or agencies to provide the best possible care for the child. For example, if a child is receiving therapy from a psychotherapist and is also receiving support from a school counsellor, it may be beneficial for the two professionals to share information about the child's progress and treatment goals. Furthermore, services such as Social Care Direct, Early Help Hubs, Family Courts, and Criminal Justice may be involved, or there may be cases where an active police investigation is taking place

Sharing data with other professionals or agencies can be beneficial for the well-being of the child, but it is important to respect the child's right to privacy and to share data only when necessary and with the appropriate consent. *And* always to keep that data specific to the necessary issue and not to include third-party information unless lawfully necessary.

Case study

Helen has been asked by the family courts to share a report on Stacey. Stacey is 12 and the victim of child sexual abuse. Police investigations are ongoing, and Helen has not informed Stacey that she is obliged to lawfully share any details about the case discussed in sessions with the criminal investigation teams/court as necessary. Stacey talks about the event with Helen and when Helen is asked to share details of the sessions, she includes the entire conversations that she has had with Stacey, which included a conversation about another girl at school that Stacey had told about the abuse.

Questions

- Do you think Helen has broken the data protection law, confidentiality, and privacy or is within the remit of an active police investigation and therefore following CPS guidelines?
- If you have not yet read these guidelines, then please head over to https://www.cps.gov.uk/legal-guidance/child-sexual-abuse-guidelines-prosecuting-cases-child-sexual-abuse.

Data breaches

Educators, practitioners, and psychotherapists should also be prepared for the possibility of a data breach, where sensitive information about a child is accidentally or intentionally accessed or disclosed without permission. This may include having a plan in place for responding to a breach and taking steps to minimise the risk of breaches occurring in the first place.

There are several steps that educators, practitioners, and psychotherapists can take to prevent data breaches when working with children. These may include implementing robust security measures, such as using secure servers and encrypting data, regularly training staff, or taking courses themselves on best practices for data security, and regularly reviewing and updating security protocols.

It is also important for educators, practitioners, and psychotherapists to be aware of the potential risks of data breaches and to take steps to mitigate them. This may include being mindful of how sensitive information is accessed and shared and ensuring that written records are kept secure. In the event of a data breach, it is important for educators and psychotherapists to have a plan in place for responding quickly and effectively. This may include informing relevant authorities, taking steps to contain the breach, and taking measures to prevent further breaches from occurring.

Case study

Alan is a trainee hypnotherapist. He is asked by his college to record the sessions he is currently undertaking for supervision in the next class. Alan has a Dictaphone and takes this into his session. He asks his client if he can record the process and the client says yes. He switches on the Dictaphone, and they conduct the session. Afterwards, Alan puts the Dictaphone into his rucksack where it sits until, he goes to his training the following week.

Questions

- What measures should Alan take to protect this data from being erased, corrupted, or accidentally played or stolen?
- If Alan was to record on his smartphone as a backup measure, what measures should also be in place there?

Children's rights

Respecting children's rights is a critical concern for educators and psychotherapists when working with children. Children have the right to be treated with dignity and respect, and it is important for professionals in these fields to be aware of and uphold those rights.

One key aspect of upholding those children's rights is ensuring that they are treated with dignity and respect. This means valuing their individual strengths and abilities and treating them with kindness and compassion. It also means recognising their inherent worth as human beings and acknowledging their right to be treated fairly and with respect, regardless of their age, abilities, or circumstances.

These rights also include the request to see their case notes, or anything else that is written about them, and this will include any notes taken about them and used in supervisory settings. In line with data protection, children also have the right to know who else writes about them and so they must be informed if the therapist's supervisors, managers, or line staff also make notes about them. When considering this, bear in mind that children over the age of 13 can request these notes and have the same rights afforded to them as other data subjects, which means that they can ask for them to be amended, changed, or deleted.

When setting out your work with children you *must* inform them of these rights, and you must document how this took place and how the child understood this conversation. It is also worth remembering that these notes can be requested for the entire time that you store these them, which brings us back to the storage limitations discussion. As a side note, it is worth bearing in mind that taking notes about children really needs to be trauma-informed and contain facts and process elements, not opinions or speculative assertions.

Again, remember that children under 13 may request their notes and parents can or may do this on their behalf. In counselling and psychotherapy settings, this can also raise ethical issues about sharing these notes – if, for example, the child is seeking a counsellor or psychotherapist without the knowledge or consent of their parent. This situation may give rise to the dilemma of whether or not you share the notes. However, third-party data will need to be redacted in these cases, unless this is a legal request, and this will require you to seek supervision and guidance from your insurance and member body in these cases.

Case study

Declan was a newly qualified practitioner. He had gained a placement with a new service for children in the local area where he lived. He worked in an office with a desk-sharing policy. One afternoon he was talking to another member of staff when they went to grab a coffee in the kitchen. His computer screen was not locked, and another member of staff was passing the desk where he sat. They saw the child's name on the screen and realised they knew this child. The member of staff did not say anything to Declan.

A few days later, Declan was called by the parent of the child who asked him how their neighbour knew that Declan was seeing their child? They were furious and demanded to know how his information had been seen by someone else? Declan could not answer this question. Declan spoke to his line manager who told him that it was probably gossip and that he hadn't done anything wrong as there were no recorded attacks on his files or computer.

Question

- What should Declan do with the information from the parent and what measures should he take to ensure that he can find out how the information he has on his computer is protected?

Case study

Louise was out in public. She used her personal phone for work clients too as she didn't want the hassle of carrying two phones. Her phone backed up to the Cloud and emails were stored on her phone as well. Louise met with her friend for coffee and as they were sitting at the table her phone, which was sitting on the table face up, rang. On the screen was the number and name of her child client with the test next to it identifying this was client number 123 (as she stored these on her computer and phone which she synced up via the Wi-Fi when she was at home). Louise's friend exclaimed: 'Oh I know that Mum, she is always in trouble with the police, I bet her kid is just the same, right?'

Questions

- What action should Louise take now her friend knows that she is seeing the child and the parent's information was visible to the friend?
- How could Louise have prevented this situation from occurring?

Case study

Megan was out shopping when her supervisor, Betty, called. She answered the phone and began taking to her supervisor. Her supervisor asked her if she could come to the office to discuss the issue she had raised as Betty could hear noise in the background. Megan said that it was fine as she was in the corner of the shopping centre and people were not near her.

Question

- What should Betty and Megan do? Should they continue the call as Megan has said she is in the corner of a shopping centre (and people were not near her)?

Legal and ethical considerations

Legal and ethical considerations are important for educators, practitioners, and psychotherapists to consider when treating children. These considerations can help to ensure that they are upholding their professional and legal obligations, and that they are providing the best possible care for the children they work with. Educators, practitioners, and psychotherapists should also be familiar with any legal or ethical guidelines related to data protection, including relevant laws and regulations and professional codes of conduct.

Legal and ethical considerations also extend to data retention and destruction practices. It is important for educators, practitioners, and psychotherapists to be familiar with any regulations or guidelines related to how long they should keep data on children, and when and how they should destroy it. Proper data retention and destruction practices help to protect the confidentiality and privacy of children and are necessary to comply with relevant laws and regulations.

Case study

Zoe was 6 years old when she saw her therapist and chiropractor for post-abuse services. Her therapist took notes about her abuse history and wrote that she thought Zoe was confabulating about certain aspects of the abuse. She wrote that Zoe was temperamental in the office and 'a bit of a madam'. The chiropractor had taken notes about Zoe and her body presentations and had kept this to the minimum standard required by the member body and insurance company stipulations. Zoe stopped seeing her therapist when she was 9 years old.

When Zoe reached 17, she was attacked at school by another student. The case went to court, and she told the solicitor that she had seen a therapist and chiropractor as a primary school child, as the injuries she sustained in the attack brought back some of her previous issues (psychologically and physically). The notes were requested by her solicitor and Zoe gave permission for them to be released. The therapist who was following her insurance company stipulations still retained Zoe's notes and was able to retrieve them. Zoe's notes had not been seen by Zoe before this point in time.

Question
• How do you think Zoe felt seeing what the therapist had written about her?

A brief review of child data protection laws and rights

There are several laws, regulations, and guidance documents that relate to data protection for children. Some examples of these include:

The General Data Protection Regulation (GDPR): This is a European Union law that applies to the processing of personal data of individuals within the EU. It sets out specific rules for protecting the personal data of children and requires that additional safeguards be put in place to protect their rights and freedoms.

The Children's Online Privacy Protection Act (COPPA): This is a United States law that applies to websites and online services that collect personal information from children under the age of 13. It requires that these websites and services obtain parental consent before collecting personal information from children and sets out specific rules for protecting the privacy of children online.

The Information Commissioner's Office (ICO) guidance on children and the GDPR: This guidance, published by the UK's data protection authority, provides specific guidance on how the GDPR applies to the processing of personal data of children and sets out best practices for protecting the privacy of children.

The United Nations Convention on the Rights of Children (UNCRC) General Comment 25 (2021): This recent change to the rights of children provides us with the knowledge that children are afforded the same rights in the online space as offline. Therefore, if you are working online, meet a child in an online space, or ask them to use digital technology with you (email, video, phone call) they have the same rights as if you were meeting them in person.

General Data Protection Regulation

The GDPR is a key piece of legislation that helps to protect the personal data of children online. It is an EU law that applies to the processing of personal data of individuals within the EU, and it sets out specific rules for protecting the personal data of children.

One of the key provisions of the GDPR is the requirement for additional safeguards to be put in place to protect the rights and freedoms of children. This means that when it comes to processing children's personal data, *additional measures must be taken to ensure that their rights are respected and that their data is protected.*

One important aspect of the GDPR when it comes to children is the requirement for parental consent. The GDPR requires that parental consent be obtained before collecting personal data from children under the age of 16 (although member states can lower this age to 13), while bearing in mind the legal definition of a child (under 18) and Gillick/Fraser case laws for the provision of certain services such as counselling. This helps to ensure that parents are aware of and can control the collection and use of their children's personal data. This would mean that children in a school counselling setting may need a special process to meet these requirements, while honouring the caveat of seeking such services that may not need parental consent. Special consideration, due diligence, and completing a Data Protection Impact Assessment may be required to assure that consent can be given by the child and how this is documented.

Please look at the mapping shown in Figure 9.1 to see the age of consent for different member states. In the UK, the age is 13 years old.[5]

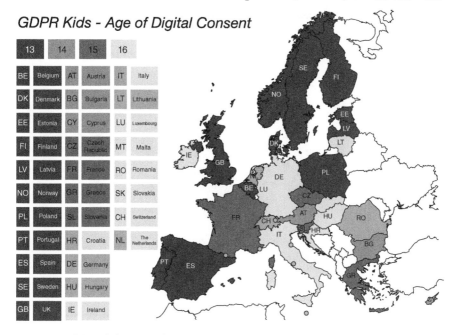

Figure 9.1 GDPR kids – age of digital consent.
Source: Image created by Elizabeth Milovidov https://www.digtalem.org for the chapter.

Another important aspect of the GDPR is the requirement for data controllers to take steps to ensure that personal data is collected and processed in a way that is appropriate for children. This includes taking into account the child's age and maturity level when designing and implementing data protection measures.

The GDPR also requires data controllers to be transparent about how they collect and use children's personal data. This means that they must provide clear and concise information about their data processing activities, including what data is being collected, why it is being collected, and how it will be used.

In addition to these requirements, the GDPR also gives children certain rights when it comes to their personal data. This includes the right to access their data, the right to have their data erased, and the right to object to the processing of their data.

An important point to note for all forms of counselling and psychotherapy services is: you are always collecting special categories of data and therefore you are required to have Data Protection Impact Assessment (DPIA) processes in place and must be able to explain to children what you do with their data, for how long, how you share this data, and for what purposes. Obtaining consent from a child requires that you adapt your contract and provide all answers to questions to ensure the child can engage in a therapeutic process with you, given their age, capacity, and understanding of data protection.

Age at which children can provide consent for the use of their personal data

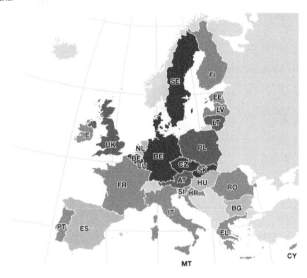

Age at which children can provide consent for the use of their presonal data

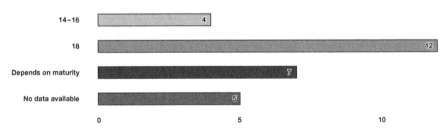

Figure 9.2 Age at which children can provide consent for the use of their personal data.
Source: Image retrieved from and copyright of http://fra.europa.eu/en/publication/2017/
mapping-minimum-age-requirements-concerning-rights-child-eu/consent-use-data-children.

Case Study

Millie is 5 years old. She is living in a separated family and Dad does not want her to speak to the counsellor in the school, he wants to seek support elsewhere. The school has a policy that a child can see the counsellor in school without parental permission. Millie's Mum has told her she can go and talk to the counsellor in school if she wants. Millie explains to the counsellor that Daddy has already found a counsellor to talk to when she visits him.

Questions

- Can the counsellors share information about Millie?
- Should the school counsellor contact Mum and Dad to discuss this?

Children'S Online Privacy Protection Act

The COPPA is a key piece of legislation that helps to protect the personal data of children online. COPPA is a United States law that applies to websites and online services that collect personal information from children under the age of 13. It requires that these websites and services obtain parental consent before collecting personal information from children and sets out specific rules for protecting the privacy of children online.

One of the key provisions of COPPA is the requirement for parental consent. COPPA requires that parental consent be obtained before collecting personal information from children under the age of 13. This helps to ensure that parents are aware of and can control the collection and use of their children's personal data.

Obtaining parental consent is not only important from a legal standpoint, but it is also an ethical requirement. It helps to ensure that children's rights are respected and that their privacy is protected; and it helps to build trust and rapport between professionals and children and their families.

COPPA also requires that websites and online services that collect personal information from children provide clear and concise information about their data collection and use practices. This includes information about what personal information is being collected, how it will be used, and with whom it will be shared.

This requirement for transparency is important for building that very trust and rapport with children and their families, and it helps to ensure that children and their parents are aware of how their personal information is being collected and used.

Case Study

Abigail is 10 years old. She does not attend school because she has anxiety and school avoidance is one of her presentations. Her mum contacts a practitioner about her daughter. The practitioner would like to talk to Abigail using Zoom or Facetime.

Questions

- Can Abigail consent to the data protection process?
- Is it okay for Abigail to use Zoom or Facetime with the practitioner?

Information Commissioner's Office

The ICO guidance on children and the GDPR are important resources for professionals working with children online. The ICO is the UK's data protection authority, and its guidance provides specific guidance on how the GDPR applies to the processing of personal data of children and sets out best practices for protecting the privacy of children.

One of the key aspects of the ICO guidance is its emphasis on the need to obtain parental consent before collecting personal data from children. The GDPR requires that parental consent be obtained before collecting personal data from children under the age of 16 (although member states can lower this age to 13), and the ICO provides further guidance on how to obtain and record parental consent.

Obtaining parental consent is not only important from a legal standpoint, but it is also an ethical requirement. It helps to ensure that children's rights are respected and that their privacy is protected, and it helps to build trust and rapport between professionals and children and their families.

The ICO guidance also provides guidance on how to ensure that personal data is collected and processed in a way that is appropriate for children. This includes taking into account the child's age and maturity level when designing and implementing data protection measures and being transparent about data collection and use practices.

In addition to these requirements, the ICO guidance also gives guidance on children's rights when it comes to their personal data. This includes the right to access their data, the right to have their data erased, and the right to object to the processing of their data.

Conclusion

Data protection is a critical concern for educators, practitioners, and psychotherapists when working with children, and, unfortunately, with rapid advances in the technological landscape, it is not always apparent how to ensure data security nor how to uphold the ethical and legal obligations. Guidance from membership bodies is seemingly absent in this area as the advances are so expansive and fast, and are growing in power and speed exponentially. Robust, appropriate training therefore must be sought outside of the normal channels of training and education to provide those educators, practitioners, and psychotherapists with the ongoing changes and strategies that they need in order to maintain their data protection and privacy practices.

Further resources

For more information on children and the law, the National Society for the Prevention of Cruelty to Children (NSPCC) provides legal summaries on several issues, including data protection and the law,[6] as well as case reviews for further insights.[7]

For information about school settings, the ICO provides examples regarding data protection as well as free lesson plans.[8]

For detailed information on children's privacy and privacy protection around the world, please consult *Children's Privacy and Safety*, International Association of Privacy Professionals (IAPP) (see Kalinda Raina, 2022).

For children's privacy and health privacy in the United States, please consult Electronic Privacy Information Center (EPIC) at epic.org, https://epic.org/issues/data-protection/childrens-privacy/.

Notes

1 See 'Information sharing: Advice for practitioners providing safeguarding services to children, young people, parents, and carers'. Accessed on 26 February 2023 at https://assets. publishing.service.gov.uk/government/uploads/system/uploads/attachment_data/file/1062969/Information_sharing_advice_practitioners_safeguarding_services.pdf.
2 'Information sharing guidance for practitioners', accessed on 26 February 2023 at https://www.ddscp.org.uk/media/derby-scb/content-assets/documents/procedures/guidance-docs/Information-Sharing-Guidance-for-Practitioners-FINAL-MAY-2019.pdf.
3 'Privacy vs confidentiality', accessed on 16 February 2023, https://www.research.uky.edu/uploads/ori-d320000-privacy-vs-confidentiality-whats-difference-pdf.
4 https://iapp.org/about/what-is-privacy/ accessed on 26 February 2023.
5 Accessed on 26 February 2023. https://ico.org.uk/for-organisations/guide-to-data-protection/key-dp-themes/children/. 'A child's personal data merits particular protection under the UK GDPR. If you rely on consent as your lawful basis for processing personal data when offering an ISS (information society service) directly to children, in the UK only children aged 13 or over are able provide their own consent. You may therefore need to verify that anyone giving their own consent in these circumstances is old enough to do so. For children under this age you need to get consent from whoever holds parental responsibility for them – unless the ISS you offer is an online preventive or counselling service.'
6 Accessed on 25 February 2023, at https://learning.nspcc.org.uk/child-protection-system/children-the-law.
7 Accessed on 25 February 2023, at https://learning.nspcc.org.uk/case-reviews.
8 Accessed on 25 February 2023, at https://ico.org.uk/for-the-public/schools/.

References and useful resources

Ayyagari, R. (2011, 30 November). ERIC – EJ971762 – Disaster at a University: A Case Study in Information Security, *Journal of Information Technology Education: Innovations in Practice*. https://eric.ed.gov/?id=EJ971762.

Children's Act (1989). Available at: https://www.legislation.gov.uk/ukpga/1989/41/contents.

EDClass (n.d.). Data breaches in education – why it's crucial to protect personal information. https://www.edclass.com/news/news-article-data-breaches-in-education-why-it-s-crucial-to-protect-personal-information.

Education and Skills Funding Agency (2022, 22 February). Record keeping and retention information for academies and academy trusts. https://www.gov.uk/government/publications/record-keeping-and-retention-information-for-academies/record-keeping-and-retention-information-for-academies-and-academy-trusts.

EPIC. https://epic.org/issues/data-protection/childrens-privacy/.

Keeping Children Safe in Education (2022). Available at https://www.gov.uk/governm ent/publications/keeping-children-safe-in-education-2.

Keeping Children Safe in Education (2023). Available at https://www.gov.uk/governm ent/publications/keeping-children-safe-in-education-2.

Livingstone, S. (2018). Children: A special case for privacy. *InterMEDIA*, *46*(2), 18–23. https://eprints.lse.ac.uk/89706/1/Livingstone_Children-a-special-case-for-privacy_ Published.pdf.

Raina, K. (2022). *Children's Privacy and Safety*. Portsmouth, NH: IAPP.

Reddy, A. (2020, 15 November). The Educator's Role: Privacy, Confidentiality, and Security in the Classroom. Student Privacy Compass. https://studentprivacycompass.org/scheid1/.

Teaching Regulation Agency (2022, 4 May). Data retention. https://www.gov.uk/gov ernment/publications/teaching-regulation-agency-data-retention/teaching-regulation-a gency-data-retention.

UNCRC (2021). General Comment 25. https://www.ohchr.org/en/documents/genera l-comments-and-recommendations/general-comment-no-25-2021-childrens-rights-relation.

Working Together to Safeguard Children (2018). Available at https://www.gov.uk/gov ernment/publications/working-together-to-safeguard-children-2.

10 Bring cyber to life

Gary Hibberd

Personal breaches: a Guide

Before we begin, it's important to know that some of the names and details in this chapter have been changed to protect the innocent and the guilty.

This chapter is intended to reflect what is happening 'in the wild'. A term that is often used in cybersecurity circles, reflecting the turbulent and often misunderstood digital landscape we live in. This chapter will not however shy away from the darker aspects of our human experience in the digital sphere. This topic is simply too important.

The book you hold has the potential to save lives. *I do not say this lightly.*

I will never forget one particular meeting with a security officer for a major government department, when I was first starting out my career in cybersecurity. In that meeting we discussed all the technical aspects of security as well as the physical elements (more on that later). As the meeting closed, I asked the officer: 'What's the worst case scenario if this data is exposed?' As the officer gathered up his papers, his response was simultaneously robust and cold: 'Someone could end up dead.' The meeting ended.

The database we were discussing held the names, addresses, dates of birth, email, and telephone details of everyone in the UK. This included the rich and famous, people on witness protection programmes, people with criminal records, and others who had left abusive relationships and started a new life elsewhere in the country.

The data was being accessed in a call centre with over 250 people, all of whom needed to be trained on the security of information. Security was at the core of what we did on a day-to-day basis, and everyone understood the responsibility that was being placed on their shoulders. In some ways, it was an easy place to instil a culture of security because everyone could understand and appreciate the relevance of security in their role.

Sadly, this often doesn't extend to our personal lives, and even more worrying is that this discipline isn't replicated in other industries.

Corporate security and protection

Would it shock you to learn that security is often seen as a necessary 'evil' for some organisations in the corporate world? Something that has to be endured and a box 'ticked' to satisfy a compliance need, such as for UK General Data Protection Regulation (GDPR, 2016) and the Data Protection Act (DPA, 2018). But as

DOI: 10.4324/9781003364184-11

a user of banks, utility companies, hospitals, schools, and universities, you surely expect them to take the security of your data seriously, right?

The good news is that many of them do. But the bad news is that, with the speed of change, the volume of data, and the number of data users only ever increasing, these corporations are fighting an arms race they can never win. Data breaches and cyberattacks are happening not just because hackers have more resources at their disposal, but because we are increasingly distracted and over-whelmed by the technology and the data we use.

This is not a chapter for statistics, so I will leave that to other writers to give you the 'logic' that backs up my emotional cry for better security. I am here to provide insight into what the real issues are, in relation to data breaches and cyberattacks.

What is personal data anyway?

Before we get into the details, we must be clear about what a data breach is. The Information Commissioner's Office (ICO) provides the following definition;

> A personal data breach means a breach of security leading to the accidental or unlawful destruction, loss, alteration, unauthorised disclosure of, or access to, per-sonal data. This includes breaches that are the result of both accidental and delib-erate causes. It also means that a breach is more than just about losing personal data. (ICO, Personal Data Breaches: https://ico.org.uk/for-organisations/report-a-breach/personal-data-breach/personal-data-breaches-a-guide/)

Notice that a breach is an event that is 'accidental' *or* 'deliberate' in nature, which means that losing a set of client notes on a bus is just as relevant as having cyber-criminals steal all your client data.

What constitutes a personal breach?

As stated above, a breach can be accidental or unlawful in nature, but what does that look like in real life? I'm going to cover some of these in more detail later by giving some real-world examples, but, for the avoidance of doubt, let's take a short walk through some of the data breaches I've witnessed in my 25 years involved in cybersecurity.

Before jumping into these examples, I would like to ask you if any of these situations has happened to you? If it has, then you have already been involved in a data breach, perhaps without even realising it. However, even if you don't think these examples apply to you, I would still urge you to ask yourself;

- What would I do?
- How would this feel to me?
- What would be the impact?

Because any one of these situations *could* happen to you, and by asking these questions as you read each scenario you will be better prepared to deal with it.

You will begin to see the gaps in your thinking and can then make a plan to close those gaps.

Access by an unauthorised third party

When a hacker manages to gain access to your computer's data files, this is clearly a data breach. In information security, we consider a data breach to be when data confidentiality, integrity, or availability is compromised. Clearly when a hacker gains access to your systems, you have no guarantee about what they have done with that data. Have they taken a copy? Have they changed any of the data, so that now the integrity (trust) in that data has gone? Or have they encrypted the data or destroyed it for their own malicious reasons? If the data are not available when needed, then this is a clear breach.

There are numerous examples of hackers gaining access to systems, stealing data, and blackmailing the company. For example, in January 2023, the UK's Royal Mail announced that they were the victim of a cyberattack where hackers had infiltrated their systems and had extracted millions of people's personal data files, and also disrupted international shipping for over two months. It left over 11,000 post offices unable to deal with international mail or parcels. Using a tool called 'LockBit', the hackers had accessed systems, encrypting them so that the Royal Mail themselves were unable to use the systems. The hackers also threatened to release the data onto the dark web – a part of the Internet that is not indexed or accessible by conventional search engines such as Google, Bing, or Yahoo – unless the Royal Mail paid a hefty ransom of over £33 million (Computer Weekly, 2023). It is called the 'dark' web because it is not visible to most Internet users and is often associated with illegal activities such as drug trafficking, arms sales, and other illicit transactions.

But it's important to keep in mind that it isn't just the big corporations that are targets of these kinds of attacks. I recall one company that called me to say that they had received a message from hackers who claimed to have stolen a copy of their entire client database. The cybercriminals were now threatening to email the customers to inform them that they had obtained a copy of the data from a weak computer system. The reputation of the company was on the line, and the criminals were 'only' asking for £1,000 in return for guarantees that they would not carry out their threat.

How is this possible? In both examples, the LockBit ransomware tool was used. LockBit isn't just a tool that hackers use – it is a service that hackers can subscribe to. This is known as 'ransomware as a service' (RaaS), and it is a clear demonstration of how criminals are now creating services to help other criminals to carry out their attacks. The RaaS allows the criminals to set the price of their ransom, and even who to target. Meaning they can select big targets (like the Royal Mail), or target millions of smaller organisations, and make smaller demands.

If you were a 'master criminal', ask yourself, what would you do? Would you target a large organisation like the Royal Mail, and demand millions? Or would you target millions of small businesses and demand just a few hundred pounds? There are risks to both, but the result is ultimately the same.

Of course, it's important to remember that even if you did pay the ransom, there are no guarantees that the criminals will give you access to your data again, or won't just release your data anyway, or won't come back and ask for more money. After all, you are dealing with criminals! Yes, you might pay your money but if they still carry out their threat, who would you complain to?

It's not just 'bad guys'

When we think of 'access by an unauthorised third-party', our minds may instinctively leap to the image of a hooded character in a basement hacking into computer systems. This is the Hollywood version of a hacker – a digital spectre to be feared and loathed for their callous nature.

But the image is only partially correct. The stereotype is that hackers wear hoodies – but they don't. Or, not always. The stereotype is that hackers work in isolation – but they don't. Due to the complex nature of many networks, they often attack a single source. In the cybersecurity industry, we term this an 'advanced persistent threat', or APT for short. When we hear this term, it means that the attackers used multiple tools or techniques to attack a target, and that often means multiple players. For those of a certain age, you might recall the TV show 'The A-Team', a band of mercenaries who were available for hire, to help solve a particular problem. Each of them had a particular skill or capability; One was the strong man, another was skilled at planning, and another was able to trick their way into a building or out of a difficult situation. This is what an APT is – skilled individuals coming together to solve a problem that no one else can solve.

But please don't be under the illusion that hackers only target large organisations. Hackers are a very real threat, but they are also always looking for easy targets. Hackers do not wake up one morning and think: 'Oh … I think today I will hack into a bank. Or maybe I'll hack into NASA [National Aeronautics and Space Administration]!' Like any common thief, they escalate from smaller crimes and smaller targets. When talking to hackers, they often speak of hacking their friends' computers, then their parents' computers, then perhaps the computers at the school or university they attend. They start simply on 'soft targets' where they know that if they get caught, the repercussions are less likely to be severe, and also where the targets' defences are likely to be easier to circumnavigate.

Ask yourself a question. If *you* were going to learn the art of hacking (and it is an art), who would you attack? The multinational organisation has a team of cyber specialists in place, monitoring a host of security controls and digital 'tripwires'. An organisation that, if breached, would bring international law enforcement agencies charging over the hill to investigate and track down the people involved. Or would you attack the small business (or practitioner) that your family uses? The one with a simple-looking website is less likely to have invested in any form of cybersecurity. The one that, should you be discovered, is unlikely to raise alarm bells with the local police force. Who would *you* attack?

It's not just hackers

We could discuss so much more, as there is a real depth to the hacker community and identity that we could explore, but that is for another time and place. But please be aware that hackers are not the only threat we have to face when thinking about the risk of personal data being accessed by unauthorised third parties.

Most of us use a cloud-based software system for accounting, banking, video conferencing, email, cloud storage, calendar management, client management, or therapy notes.

My question to you is: What does it say within the terms and conditions of using that service about the company's employees (or third parties) accessing the data that you are storing there?

In some respects, you could argue that because you have signed-up to their terms of business, they are indeed 'authorised', and therefore no breach has occurred. But how does that sit with you when, for example, you are holding a one-to-one video therapy session?

Are you comfortable in the knowledge that the video conferencing company have access to the recorded sessions? Are you happy that a member of staff could listen in to your sessions at any time 'to improve customer experience'? Would that be classified as unauthorised?

For the avoidance of doubt, the vast majority of commercially available video conferencing services, like Zoom and Microsoft Teams do exactly this. In a blog post by Microsoft, in April 2020, they discussed the matter of privacy and security in Microsoft Teams, stating, 'We take strong measures to ensure access to your data is restricted and carefully define requirements for responding to government requests for data' (Microsoft, 2020).

At no point do they say: 'We do not allow access to your data.' It is simply 'restricted'. Please note that I am not saying that these platforms are not secure. For example, Microsoft state that they meet more than 90 regulatory and industry security standards (Microsoft, n.d., 'Managing compliance in the cloud').

But secure does not mean private. Therefore, unless you are being very transparent with your clients that their data may be accessed by a third party such as Zoom or Microsoft, they are not authorised – and this could be classified as a data breach.

In the early days of the pandemic, video-conferencing tools became extremely popular and were, in some cases quite literally, a lifesaver for individuals and businesses alike. It is hard to imagine what the pandemic would have looked like if this technology had not existed. We were able to stay connected to friends, family, loved ones, and customers and clients, which helped many of us to survive. But with this technology came the ability for people to gain access to conferencing calls, as session IDs became known and shared among wider groups. When this began to happen, 'Zoom-bombing' became a very real and present risk, where an uninvited guest would appear in a meeting and play loud music or show a disturbing video or images in order to disrupt the event. These people became known as 'disrupters', because that was their intent, or at least that is what we know was their intent.

Very quickly, video-conferencing tools had to improve their security, and began including password-protected sessions and 'waiting rooms' to prevent these disrupters from gaining access to a session. But it's no surprise that many of these security features are not enabled as standard. Why? Because doing so can make them a little harder to use, and therefore may impact on the 'customer experience'. Therefore, they leave it to you and me to enable passwords, waiting rooms, and other security features. The message is clear – the responsibility to protect ourselves is ours.

Sending personal data to an incorrect recipient

Have you ever sent an email to the wrong person? To be honest, most of us have. Email systems have made the job of sending emails easier by helpfully completing an email address even when you only type in the first letters of a name. Start typing an email to 'Ga...' and the options will be 'Gary...', 'Gail...', 'Gareth', etc.

According to some digital commentators, we send over 319 billion emails every day, so is it any wonder we send the odd email to the wrong person? If the email in question doesn't contain any sensitive information, then what's the harm? But what if the email contains the written notes of a recent therapy session or confidential meeting? Then the impact could be far more damaging to you, your reputation, and to the data subject.

It's important to state at this point that data also exist in physical form. Consider the following example.

When Steve answered the door to the neighbour, he wasn't expecting to be handed an envelope full of his medical records. The neighbour sheepishly explained that the letter had been sent to the wrong address, and how he had opened the letter without thinking. The letter was clearly addressed to Steve, but the address number was transposed, from '21' to '12'.

Steve stared at the envelop as the neighbour explained that he had also been expecting a large document through the post, so it was only upon opening it and reviewing some of the content he realised he wasn't the intended recipient.

Steve felt the anxiety rise from the pit of his stomach. Anxiety that he had held at bay for some considerable time, through a mix of therapy and prescribed medication. All of which was detailed in the medical records his friendly neighbour was handing him.

There was no way of knowing whether the neighbour had read any or all of the files. They gave no impression that they had, but Steve's anxiety was such that it left him with the same feelings of despair and isolation that he had fought so long to conquer.

Over subsequent months, he convinced himself that the neighbour's cheery disposition and occasional glances were evidence that his 'dark secret' was now the talk of the neighbourhood. It was a feeling he just couldn't shake.

It took a full six months for Steve to put his house on the market, and move out of the area. It forced a change in school for his children, and caused considerable disruption to his partner who, while being supportive, couldn't dissuade him from the paranoia that had taken hold.

The emotional distress was caused by a simple, and highly preventable data input error.

Computing devices containing personal data being lost or stolen

Our digital assistants go with us everywhere. On trains, to meetings, therapy sessions, schools, hospitals, the local park, restaurants, pubs, clubs, bedrooms, and even the toilet. Knowing that you carry around a mini-computer, you'd think people would take more care of these expensive and highly valuable devices. Not because the device is costly, but because the information they contain is often priceless.

Computing devices include mobile phones, tablets, laptops, and desktop computers. Many of us use a mix of one or more of these items on a daily basis to access everything from therapy notes to our shopping and online banking services. These devices carry a plethora of personal data related to ourselves, let alone the people we interact with. They often contain photos, videos, messages, and emails relating to everything from sexual encounters to our latest electricity bill.

Despite the sensitive nature of these devices, we blithely carry them around in the bottom of a bag, or leave them on a desk or a bar, just begging to be picked up or left behind.

This was the situation that faced a young therapist who, following a particularly long day at a school, working with a number of children, left to meet her partner in a bar in the centre of town. As the bus took her into the heart of the city, she emailed her colleagues a brief update, sent a text to her partner, and dozed uneasily as she recalled the sessions and considered what needed to be done. Upon arriving at the bar, she had a much needed warm welcome and a cold drink waiting for her. Her partner listened without comment as she relayed the details of her day, omitting any personal details for fear of being overheard.

The evening conversation relaxed and as the conversation flowed, so did the wine as the bar became busier. It was dark before they left the bar and headed back to the car. Her partner unlocked the car and as they settled into their seats, she reached into her coat pocket to check her phone.

But her phone was gone. She frantically checked her pockets and bag, but it wasn't there. Dashing back to the bar she returned to the table they had been sitting at, which was now occupied by a group of people, none of whom had seen her phone. She asked at the bar, but it hadn't been handed in.

It was gone.

Her device contained:

- Banking details
- Credit card details
- Email accounts – both personal and work
- Shopping accounts
- Social media accounts

- Personal photos and videos
- Discount cards
- Personal contact details
- Client contact details
- Personal appointments
- Therapy appointments (including names and contact details)
- Therapy notes (including recorded sessions).

What is the impact of cybercrime and data breaches?

Let us be clear; Cybercrime, or criminal activity that is committed using the Internet or other forms of computer networks, can have serious and harmful consequences for individuals, businesses, and society.

One way that cybercrime harms people is through financial loss. For example, individuals may fall victim to online scams and fraud, such as phishing attacks or unauthorised charges on their credit cards. Businesses may suffer financial losses as a result of cyberattacks that disrupt their operations or steal sensitive financial information. These types of cybercrimes can result in significant financial losses for the victims and can be particularly devastating for those who are already struggling financially.

Another way that cybercrime harms people is through the theft and misuse of or data breaches of their personal information. Hackers may access and steal sensitive personal information, such as Social Security or National Insurance numbers, addresses, passwords, medical records, and financial information, which can be used for identity theft or other nefarious purposes. The consequences of this type of cybercrime can be long-lasting and severe, as victims may have to deal with the financial and emotional toll of identity theft for years to come.

Cybercrime can also harm people by disrupting their daily lives and causing stress and anxiety. For example, ransomware attacks, in which hackers hold a person's computer or device hostage until a ransom is paid, can be particularly disruptive and stressful. Similarly, online harassment and stalking can have serious psychological effects on the victims, as they may feel constantly threatened or unsafe.

In addition to harming individuals, cybercrime can also have negative consequences for businesses, institutions (such as universities), and society. Businesses may suffer significant financial losses as a result of cyberattacks, and they may also experience damage to their reputation and customer trust. This can lead to a decline in business and financial stability. Cybercrime can also have broader societal consequences, as it may undermine trust in online systems and technologies, and it may also lead to increased regulation and restrictions on Internet use.

Overall, cybercrime and data breaches have the potential to cause significant harm to individuals, businesses, and society. It is important for individuals and organisations to take steps to protect themselves and their sensitive information, and for law enforcement agencies to work to identify and prosecute those who engage in cybercrime or allow data breaches to occur.

What does the law say?

The laws that govern personal data protection are the General Data Protection Regulation and, in the UK, the Data Protection Act 2018. It is surprising to me how many people have heard of the GDPR but very few have actually read it. This is like saying that the Harry Potter books confuse you – because you've never read them!

Obviously the GDPR and the Data Protection Act are never going to be as entertaining or universally loved as Harry Potter, but I feel the general confusion comes from a lack of exposure to these important laws. And remember – they are laws. These are not 'nice to have', or 'guidance to follow'. They are laws that relate to how we must control and process data. They are as relevant to you and your business as health, safety, and tax laws.

Although this chapter is not a deep exploration into what these laws say, I think we need to be clear about what they say about what a personal data breach actually is.

According to Recital 85 of the GDPR a personal data breach may:

> if not addressed in an appropriate and timely manner, result in physical, material or non-material damage to natural persons such as loss of control over their personal data or limitation of their rights, discrimination, identity theft or fraud, financial loss, unauthorised reversal of pseudonymisation, damage to reputation, loss of confidentiality of personal data protected by professional secrecy or any other significant economic or social disadvantage to the natural person concerned.
>
> (ICO, p. 66)

Clearly a breach can have a range of adverse effects on individuals, which include emotional distress, and physical and material damage. It is true that some personal data breaches will not lead to risks beyond the inconvenience to those who need the data to do their job. However, other breaches put people at significant risk and may affect individuals in very real ways.

Reporting a breach

Section 85 of the GDPR goes on to say that, as soon as a controller becomes aware that a personal data breach has occurred, the controller should notify the personal data breach to the supervisory authority (in the UK, this is the ICO) without undue delay and, where feasible, not later than 72 hours after having become aware of it. The only reason for not notifying them is if the controller is able to demonstrate that the personal data breach is unlikely to result in a risk.

The controller in the therapist/patient scenario is the therapist, as they are the ones who determine the purpose and the kind of data that will be processed. Sharing the data with a third-party platform (such as a Cloud-based system) makes them a 'processor'.

So, be under no illusion – the controller *is* the therapist. And you cannot outsource your responsibility or accountability for the protection of personal data.

It's all fine, right?

I'm not going to focus on the fines that could be levied against you or your business for a breach, or the enforcement notices that could prevent you from practising. But we do need to remember that fines and claims for compensation are very real possibilities in the wake of a data breach.

Compensation claims can be made on the basis of material or non-material damages. Material damages include any financial losses the data subject may experience due to the breach. For example, in the event of identity theft, the claimant may seek compensation for any monies lost. Where there are claims for non-material damage, the claimant may seek compensation for any emotional distress or mental health issues related to the data breach. For example, if they have increased feelings of anxiety or stress due to the breach of their data, then there is a good case for compensation to be paid.

Claims for compensation and fines that can be levied can be substantial, but, in truth, the amount of money you are realistically going to be fined is relatively low. Perhaps a few hundred pounds, or even a few thousand, might be the only financial impact you receive.

However, it's important to note that the impact of a breach might also extend to an impact on your reputation, and in fact it is the reputational damage that worries people the most. In many organisations, large or small, the biggest risk or threat is that a breach may lead to a loss of customer or client trust. After all, your clients have shared their private data with you thinking you have put in place all the necessary technical, organisational, and physical controls to protect them.

Does this seem unreasonable? What about you? When was the last time you checked with your bank to ask about their security? Or the online shop? Or the gym you visit? What about the doctor? You have assumed they are taking appropriate steps to protect your data, so why should you be different? What are *you* doing to protect people?

But the fear of fines should not be the reason we implement good security and put in place prudent controls to ensure data protection and privacy. The reason should be, because we understand the impact a breach has, or can potentially have, on real people. We need to hear about real incidents that have had real-world impact for both the practitioners and their clients (and sometimes both). What I am going to emphasise is the impact that a breach has on the individual and reveal just how bad it can get.

Make no mistakes, in the stories we share here, I am holding nothing back, and this is not sensationalised to make a point. There are other, far darker recesses of the Internet where the stories are beyond the scope of this book, and should only be shared in an environment where the situation and our reactions can be carefully monitored and cared for. There is a duty of care here, and I have provided stories that I believe illuminate the central point, without being sensational or voyeuristic.

But please be under no illusion, the issues and ramifications related to data breaches and incidents that cybersecurity and data protection specialists like me see on a day-to-day basis is nothing short of shocking.

The stories you are about to read are real. The details have been changed to protect the innocent and the guilty. What I ask of you is to put yourself in the position of the affected individual and ask yourself:

- 'What would I do differently?'
- 'How would I feel if *my* data had been exposed?'
- 'Is there anything I could have done to prevent this?'

Breach example #1

When travelling on a train Adi enjoyed the silence and solitude it offered, allowing him to focus on the task at hand. As a counsellor, Adi understood the importance of capturing the meeting notes in a format that would allow him to refer back to previous sessions, quickly and easily.

With headphones on, the world flew by in a blur to the Harry Potter soundtrack, as written text and information become more structured on the screen.

It wasn't long, however, before Adi's eyes began to droop. It had been a long day, and with the work, music, and the steady rhythmic motion of the carriage, it wasn't long before Adi's eyes closed and sleep beckoned.

In what felt like only seconds, Adi felt the train's pace begin to slow as the train conductor announced the imminent arrival at Sheffield – Adi's stop! In a flurry, Adi began gathering up the papers, laptop, charger, coat, and bag and headed off the train.

Breathlessly standing on the concourse, Adi clasped the bag tight and headed for the taxi rank, and the final leg of the journey home.

Weeks later ...

Adi knew that the notebook was missing and that the notes from the London trip had gone. Recalling the journey home, Adi had reconciled himself to the fact that it either was left on the train or in the taxi. Either way, it was gone. Nothing could be done now.

It was almost out of Adi's mind when a call from an irate client came through. They started by asking for an explanation of how their details could have been left on a train! And why hadn't they been informed? It transpired that the notebook had been picked up by another passenger, who dutifully handed it in. The train company reviewed the content of the notebook, were able to establish a contact name and details from the pages, and had spoken to one of Adi's clients and alerted them to the fact that their personal data had been left on a train.

They hadn't contacted Adi, because Adi hadn't thought to include 'In case of loss' contact details. The client was understandably furious and promptly reported Adi to the Information Commissioners Office. In the weeks that followed, and following numerous calls and emails to the ICO, and sleepless nights, the ICO upheld the complaint against Adi, who was ordered to pay £1,400 to the claimant and instructed to amend working practices and processes to reduce the likelihood of a breach in future.

Data = people

It's all too easy to forget that information we collect relates to real, living, breathing people. We hear of a data breach involving hundreds, thousands, and even millions of 'data points', but forget that each one is a data 'subject'. A real person with real lives who can be harmed in very real ways.

For example, it should go without saying that therapists have access to some of the most sensitive information in existence. It *should* go without saying, but I find myself repeating this mantra far too frequently.

Consider for a second the banking sector, which is heavily regulated and legislated to ensure data security is in place. But the financial sector (largely) only has access to our financial records. They know what you've spent, when, and how often. They know your credit rating and therefore your capability to repay a loan (or not). Of course, financially motivated criminals are going to target the banking sector and individual bank accounts to separate us from our hard-earned money. The financial sector invests millions, and often billions, of pounds/dollars in keeping this data safe, and where they don't there are significant legislative costs to pay.

But it's just money. The impact on an individual when money is lost is of course significant, and can lead to financial hardship, negative credit ratings, and, in the most severe cases, loss of income or status.

But it's still just money. The financial sector is now geared up for financial losses due to data breaches and cybercrime. Customers (you and I) carry this cost in increased banking charges, which means that the only loser is you and me in the event of a data breach or scam.

But it's still just money. The information that a therapist processes is deeply and profoundly personal. Patients reveal their deepest, darkest fears or experiences. With careful guidance they reveal, in great detail, thoughts and desires that they can't share with their life partner or family for fear of what the impact might be.

Therapists have a duty of care to 'do no harm', yet, when asked about cyber-security and data protection, it is often less than convincing that they are giving data protection due care and attention.

But what's the worst that could happen?

Breach example #2

Clients put their trust in a therapy company to keep their notes and diagnoses private. Then the ransom demands start to arrive. Back in 2018 this was the situation that people faced in Finland.

Jose's blood ran cold as he re-read the email that was sitting quietly on his computer screen. The mouse somehow pointing directly at the word 'Bitcoin', a word he had heard of before but never really understood much about. The email read:

> We are in possession of information obtained from Vastaamo, a company that provides psychotherapy services to therapists.

If we do not receive €200 worth of Bitcoin within 24 hours, this will increase to €500 and after 48, to €600. If we do not receive payment your information will be released and sent to your friends, employer and on the web.

If payment is received, your information will be permanently deleted from our servers. Here is a link to instructions on how to purchase Bitcoin. A helpline has been established, so please call this number if you need support.

Jose didn't know what to do, but felt he had limited option but to pay for the Bitcoin. But before this he decided to contact his therapist.

Following numerous emails and telephone voice messages, the therapist called to explain that unfortunately the breach was real. They explained that Vastaamo had announced a significant data breach a few days earlier. It transpired that a security flaw in the company's IT systems had exposed their entire patient data-base to the open Internet – not just email addresses and Social Security numbers, but the actual written notes that therapists had taken.

Like sharks circling in the ocean, hackers are constantly on the look-out for exposed data, and just like blood in the ocean, once they sense it is vulnerable, they will attack.

Jose had been to see the therapist to discuss an ongoing alcohol dependency, which was largely the result of traumatic childhood experiences and events that had only recently surfaced following the death of a family member. The thought of this information ever becoming public hadn't even crossed his mind. Afterall, Jose had only told one person and that person was bound by some kind of oath, right? They wouldn't reveal the contents of their discussions?

Perhaps not. But the therapist was indeed revealing Jose's inner most thoughts and feelings. They were sharing them with Vastaamo, a third-party, Cloud software provider. The data was stored in the Cloud, and accessible by the therapist from anywhere in the world. All they needed to access their client data was the appropriate login details, or for a flaw to exist, which meant that anyone, in the entire world, could access the information.

Hundreds of people received the same email that Jose had received. Hundreds of people were now having to make the conscious decision to either pay the ransom or run the risk of having their sessions revealed to their work colleagues, friends, family, and life partners.

But surely the company, Vastaamo, took precautions and protected the data? How could this happen? The truth is, there is no such thing as 100 per cent secure. The more complex a system, the more likelihood there is a security flaw or gap. It's like building a house – the bigger the house, the more pipes and wiring, and the more windows and doors you need. All of which need to be maintained and managed on an ongoing basis. Now turn that house into a multi-storey sky-scraper with people coming in and out at all times of the day and you begin to see the size of the problem.

But none of this mattered to Jose. He had a sleepless night that began to pull at the very insecurities that he had gone to see his therapist about in the first place. With the threat of having his data revealed, he decided to pay the ransom and buy the Bitcoin. The process was remarkably simple and even when he struggled a little with the 'digital wallet', the number he obtained from the hackers was serviced by a polite lady who walked him through the process of paying the €500.

At the end of the transaction, he was told his data would be erased and he would not be contacted again. And for him, this is where the story ends. Except it isn't …

Jose knows there is a real possibility that the cybercriminals will come back and demand more money. With the threat of having his details revealed he has returned to the substance abuse about which he had originally been to see the therapist.

He doesn't feel he is able to see a therapist, as the trust in that community is no longer there.

Conclusion

Cybercrime and data breaches are now a fact of life. Although we can do our best to reduce their impact or likelihood, the truth is that we must constantly be vigilant to both their prevention and presence. This is not to say that being a victim of cybercrime or having a breach is inevitable. I do not subscribe to the notion that everyone is going to be a victim or that everyone will one day be the cause of a breach.

I am saying that unless we take due care and pay attention, the likelihood of us suffering a breach or becoming victims is increasing exponentially. Like it or not, we are all connected by the digital networks we use, and we all have a digital footprint. In business there is a saying that 'data is more valuable than gold' – and it's true. There is not a business or institution in the land that does not need or thrive from data. The more data available, the more information can be obtained, and the more intelligence and knowledge can be used. The more we use technology, the deeper our footprint becomes. So, what can we do about it?

It is worth keeping in mind that our digital super-highway is very similar to the highways we use to travel around in our physical world. They are both becoming highly congested, and the more we use them the more vigilant and careful we need to be. No one is suggesting that, because the roads are busier, you're guaranteed to have an accident. But if you take your eyes off the road, even for a moment, the likelihood of an accident vastly increases.

When it comes to our travels on the super-highway, we need to ask whether we need safer vehicles or safer drivers. I believe the answer to this question is – we need both.

References and useful resources

Computer Weekly (2023). Royal Mail branches still struggling after cyber attack. https://www.computerweekly.com/news/365530230/Royal-Mail-branches-still-struggling-after-cyber-attack#:~:text=Royal%20Mail%20has%20successfully%20restored,they%20have%20bought%20postage%20online.

Data Protection Act (2018). Legislation. https://www.legislation.gov.uk/ukpga/2018/12/contents/enacted.

EU General Data Protection Regulation (2016). https://commission.europa.eu/law/law-topic/data-protection_en

ICO (n.d.). Disclosure, page 66. https://ico.org.uk/media/about-the-ico/disclosure-log/2014536/irq0680151-disclosure.pdf.

ICO (n.d.). Personal data breaches. https://ico.org.uk/for-organisations/guide-to-data-protection/guide-to-the-general-data-protection-regulation-gdpr/personal-data-breaches/.

ICO (n.d.). Section 85, GDPR. https://ico.org.uk/media/about-the-ico/disclosure-log/2014536/irq0680151-disclosure.pdf.

Microsoft (n.d.). Compliance in the cloud. https://www.microsoft.com/en-us/trust-center/compliance/compliance-overview.

Microsoft (n.d.). Our commitment to privacy and security in Microsoft Teams. https://news.microsoft.com/en-my/2020/04/08/our-commitment-to-privacy-and-security-in-microsoft-teams/.

Zoom bombing. https://dictionary.cambridge.org/dictionary/english/zoombombing.

11 Conclusion and top tips

Catherine Knibbs

Conclusion and top tips for practitioners

A conclusions is usually the last chapter of a book that sums up the topic as a reflection. A chapter where you can essentially see the highlights and main points of the story or theory. Given the book has encapsulated several professional sectors, however, it can be difficult to summarise this into one or two coherent paragraphs without saying that *data protection is your practice from beginning to end*. In order to do this, you are going to need to read the advice and guidance in this book to provide you with the skills and understanding as to why, how, when, and where you need to protect data, and this includes your own data, by the way, as the whole message of this book is likely to leave you questioning what other people do with your data. Perhaps this never crossed your mind before now, or was a thought on the road to learning about looking after other people's data. Little did you think that you might just find yourself talking like Cath and Gary and asking companies about *their* policies and procedures!

As such the following tips here are handed out at the end of the training, or discussed in training that both Cath and Gary have been involved in during the early days of the General Data Protection Regulation (GPDR), when the world felt like we were speaking to people who had lost their heads. Cath has spent many years with counselling organisations discussing various aspects of online safety and the trauma of not protecting clients' data, because, as you will have seen in this book, you may not even know there is a problem until it happens.

At many events, when Cath challenges existing practices it is to help the various organisations, membership bodies, and individuals oversee how their behaviour with and use of technology can put them and the data they hold at risk; and to help them see how they need guidance on these topics in more than simplistic forms or quick webinars to wholly understand the expertise needed – and as presented in this book. It is a shame that this book does not have all the issues discussed in the form of case studies, nor can we know at this time all the issues that have taken place during the period of lockdown, where systems were used that were not secure. As this book was going to print there was a very large breach taking place of a US-based service (also used by

DOI: 10.4324/9781003364184-12

some UK practitioners). It had been selling the data on the registered users and their clients to those dark web spaces that Gary alluded to in Chapter 10. This service was not under the UK or EU laws and people were 'sold out' for what might have been pennies for what could be a lifetime of misery.

When they do training, both Gary and Cath say, no matter who the training is for: this is a horror story based on reality. This is not 'sensationalism', as Cath has been told on many occasions for telling these stories, this could be a matter of life or death. And the most difficult aspect of that is that the professional may well be the one to feel the burden of responsibility for that, because they didn't know and didn't get the training.

People often ask what service can deliver security, cybersecurity, data protection, privacy, confidentiality, child protection, and online safety and tie this into the professions of health and wellbeing?

Cath put together an organisation called Privacy4 to do this very thing in 2018 and created online training using almost every person in this book as the consultants who gave their time and expertise to help design that course. The fact is, at the start of lockdown over 250 people signed up for a free business continuity plan that Gary provided, a contract for online work (by Cath), and some live video meetings were given out for free. In the statistical analysis that followed, not one person completed the course and 4 per cent was the highest completion rate for the 240 people who signed up. GDPR scares people, so though I can imagine reading this book might have cemented that idea further, it might also have provided a guiding light showing that data protection is not that bad once you understand it.

In the process of creating this book and speaking with Meg Moss (Foreword) over a number of years, Privacy4 provided the National Counselling Society (soon changing its name to National Counselling and Psychotherapy Society) with some online training for practitioners to do in their own time. You can head to their website to take this course if you wish to have a continuing professional development certificates (see https://counsellingcpd.org/courses/privacy4/).

This book is a template for you, but it is not a course. The essential guide that Gary and Cath put together (www.privacy4.co.uk) is exactly that but it is not training. Discursive elements and real-life examples need to be in a room of people where specificity can be unpicked and conversations can take place about what data are, what services do, and how they serve those they work with. I hope this can now become less alarming to think about and welcomed into the profession as part of the training route and as compulsory as ethics and safeguarding.

As we say at Privacy4: *Know the Law!*

Warmly,

Catherine

Here are 10 top tips from Privacy4 Training:

Tasks post-training.

Don't panic this is a process not a destination.

1 Register with the ICO (processing of special categories of data require you to do so).
2 Buy good Internet security software.
3 Commit to and complete your Data Protection Impact Assessment.
4 Read all the privacy policies of third-party software (e.g. your antivirus provider, your email system, your operating system).
5 Create a new privacy policy for your customers and clients to communicate the above.
6 If you don't understand the third-party privacy policies, communicate this to your customers and clients when you give them a privacy policy of your own. Be transparent and allow them to make a choice about their communication with you.
7 Use a specified platform for the purposes of your trade or profession. For example, confidential services require data to be kept within the UK and EU (so do not use US-based systems unless you can convey to your customers and clients *all* the risks associated with data being processed under US law. *Hint*: Under US law, they don't have data protection laws so can use the data they collect for any purposes.)
8 Communicate with your member or trade body about your data and find out where they keep your records and for how long, etc.
9 If you share your data with companies (e.g. solicitors, schools, employee assistance providers (EAPs)) ask the same questions as above.
10 Request the GDPR policy of any services you provide your services to, e.g. schools, clinics, etc. so you can assess if you are a joint controller.

Keep up to date with changes, read the GDPR and DPA 2018

Tips for practitioners, by Kim Page

1 Assemble your own data points. Learn from the inside out by following your own workflows.
2 Make tech your friend. Discuss with peers and search for new ideas, ways of working. Also stay close to any method of reporting scams or poor tech practice.
3 Lead the way, one step at a time. Diarise a tech assessment every quarter.

4 Give clients the gift of privacy. Be able to work with them without them needing to sign up to any third party.
5 Showcase your ethical practice. Tell future clients that you take tech seriously and have taken steps to provide them with a safe space online.
6 Check how you are connecting to any businesses as well as with clients. Data points can hide here too!
7 Update your kit. Get the best you can afford. As software improves it relies on the most up-to-date operating systems and your kit needs to be able to handle these – *especially* for security. Three years is a good timeframe to aim for.
8 Look for as few a number of software services as possible. And choose them yourself, rather than letting clients choose.
9 Walk a mile in your client's shoes. Keep a watchful eye on all the routes a customer can use to find you and communicate with you.
10 Use practice management software, built for therapists and counsellors and no one else.

Index

Italic page numbers indicate figures.

Printed and bound by CPI Group (UK) Ltd, Croydon, CR0 4YY

07/08/2024

01024371-0012